SAME
TIME
NEXT
WEEK

True Stories of Working
Through Mental Illness

Edited by
LEE GUTKIND

Introduction by
PETER D. KRAMER

Foreword by
KAREN WOLK FEINSTEIN

InFACT
BOOKS

Tom Mallouk's "I'm Not a Noun Either" is excerpted
and adapted from "Reflections on Psychiatry, the
Fear of Insanity, Trauma and Psychotherapy,"
originally published in the Spring 2014 issue of
Solstice, and appears here by permission of the
author.

Requests for permission to reproduce material
from this work should be sent to:

    Rights and Permissions
    In Fact Books
    c/o Creative Nonfiction Foundation
    5501 Walnut Street, Suite 202
    Pittsburgh, PA 15232

Cover and text design by Heidi Roux

ISBN: 978-1-937163-19-8

CONTENTS

WHAT WORKS WHEN NOTHING HAS WORKED?

Peter D. Kramer

Disorders of mind and brain can be powerful. Something goes wrong. The glitch or, worse, major disturbance may involve reasoning, perception, feeling, energy, relationship patterns, personality traits, or repeated behaviors. The problems rarely remain delimited. They can claim much of a life, unless a solution emerges. Sometimes, after years of slippage—intrusive thoughts, destructive impulses, paralyzing mood states, relentless addiction, intractable pain—a person finds a footing. But how? What works when nothing has worked?

These memoirists, whether healers or sufferers, are mostly in agreement: relief comes from outside the mainstream of care. It's not that there are no good guys; in "What Would My Mother Say?" Annita Sawyer—once suicidal and hallucinating—writes of "a psychiatrist whose steady centeredness, flexibility, and sense of humor got through to me." But Sawyer's story is also one of institutional failure: over-aggressive treatment, grounded in a failure to explore, to listen, to elicit the crucial elements of history and experience.

Most often in these stories of recovery, the source of change is idiosyncratic, unexpected, a step or two off the common path.

Standard-issue treatments garner scant respect. Cognitive behavioral therapy, the current darling of the professions, is no favorite. It's the existential approach—personal presence, radical acceptance—that does the job, if the job can be done through psychotherapy.

Unconventional moves in psychotherapy receive the occasional nod—holding, walking, digging a hole to bury misery and shame. Generally, the cure is partial. That's fine, too. The first goal, when people are drowning, is to get them afloat. Reaching shore comes later.

Medication earns mixed reviews. Ronald Bassman, a patient turned psychotherapist, finds them overused: "Research has shown that these drugs do physical damage and inhibit recovery." J. Timothy Damiani, a psychiatrist, works a one-off transformation with lithium, a drug that's on my own short list of favorites.

And what if, as is mostly the rule here, mainstream efforts—talk therapy and drugs—are not enough? We learn about religious retreat, reading, speech therapy, self-advocacy, and the kindness of relatives, friends, and fellow patients. For Candy Schulman's brother-in-law, Will, laid low by an especially debilitating form of schizophrenia, the miracle arrives mostly on its own, spontaneous remission nudged along, perhaps, by modest help from medication.

One villain in these tales is diagnosis. Patients accumulate labels, with little clarity gained. Some of these labels are mistaken; more are unhelpful. Reading Sharron Hoy's account of her long-term misdiagnosis, I was reminded of a lecture by my colleague George Vaillant, titled "The Beginning of Wisdom Is Never Calling a Patient a Borderline." Certain categories lead us, doctors and patients both, deeper into the thicket.

As a practicing psychiatrist, I worry, if slightly, that this collection obscures the reliable help available from routine care.

What with scandals concerning doctors and drug companies and controversy concerning diagnosis and the role of placebo effects, the media sometimes convey the impression that the mental health professions have little to offer.

In practice, most patients who seek treatment respond to it. To cite a snippet of data from the field I know most about, mood disorders, a well-conducted Swedish study found that when primary care doctors offered moderately depressed patients standard medication, 90 percent of those who followed through experienced substantial improvement. *Why* is a different matter—perhaps the white coat did the job; perhaps (I hold this view) antidepressants are reasonably effective. The point is that typical patients with common ailments generally do well.

Diagnosis, too, can be decisive. Psychiatry and psychology have specific approaches, pharmacologic and psychotherapeutic, for obsessive-compulsive disorder, bipolar disorder, and others. And then there is the boundary with general medicine. Epilepsy, anemia, hormone or vitamin deficiencies, side effects of prescribed drugs—the list of categories for which specific remedies exist is a long one. Often, fixing or mitigating the underlying condition relieves the mental symptoms decisively.

Still, the professions' failures are legion. Physicians, psychologists, nurses, social workers, and psychotherapists of many stripes—we all work with non-responders, with people who suffer what is sometimes called the career of depression, the career of anorexia, the career of schizophrenia, and on and on. Chronicity and recurrence are the norm. These stories come from that territory, bleak and fascinating. What is the route across, the passage through, the fruitful journey? Confidence and curiosity on the part of caregivers make a difference. So do compassion and persistence on the part of coworkers and employers, ministers and fellow sufferers, friends and relations. But those answers, true in their way, are too pat. These detailed personal accounts point to the limit of our art and science. When they no longer avail, we are fully in the realm of what used also to be called the existential: where terror prevails, where stubbornness and belated good luck become critical, where the individual, hand-crafted solution is the only one we can hope to find.

....

Peter D. Kramer is a psychiatrist and author, and currently a clinical professor of psychiatry and human behavior at Brown University. His books include Listening to Prozac *and* Against Depression.

OVERCOMING INSTITUTIONAL FAILURE

Lee Gutkind

In some ways, the subtitle of this book—*Working Through Mental Illness*—doesn't quite capture the challenge, struggle, and triumph of these remarkable true stories. There's more—a reality Peter Kramer captures in his incisive and thought-provoking introduction when he refers to the inadequate and sometimes harmful treatment of those who suffer from mental illness and to an "institutional failure" which, I believe, is at the heart of the problem.

I have been writing about the world of mental health for most of my career, focusing primarily on this "institutional failure"—the dysfunctional system that inadequately supports and often significantly harms patients and their families and, indirectly, our entire country. The statistics are staggering and sobering. According to the National Institute of Mental Health, one in four adults (approximately 61.5 million Americans) and one in five young persons (ages 13–18) experiences a diagnosable mental disorder in a given year. Even more staggering, 60 percent of those adults and half of those adolescents and young adults will not receive treatment over a year's period. Besides being morally indefensible, this is practically unsustainable. Serious mental illness costs America nearly $200 billion in lost earnings every year. And the societal stigma attached to those who have suffered from mental illness makes recovery and reintegration into society—and the workforce—challenging and sometimes impossible.

Patients and their families are not the only victims of this institutional failure. Mental health professionals—including psychiatrists, psychologists, nurses, and social workers—are in the front line, often struggling to overcome the inadequacies and the corruption of the system. They are, more often than not, underpaid and overworked and, consequently, pressured to deal with patients and families in an assembly line fashion—that is, if time, availability, and resources permit treatment at all. In our current system, even patients and families with extensive insurance coverage are often unable to spend time with therapists on a regular basis.

Despite their vital importance, there's an incredible and growing scarcity of psychiatrists in this country. According to the US Department of Health and Human Services, in more than half the nation's 3,100 counties, there are no practicing psychiatrists, psychologists, or social workers. Psychiatry is one of the lowest paid of all of the medical specialties. Master's degree social workers (MSWs), who are responsible for most therapy and contact with patients and families, are often paid less than factory workers.

And yet, despite all of these barriers, many who have suffered from mental illness—even the most heinous of diagnoses—somehow survive, recover, find work, rejoin loved ones, and live meaningful and productive lives. Often, the help of a good and devoted therapist, combined with carefully prescribed medication, is essential to this process. The encouraging and vitally important message of the true stories collected here is that a diagnosis of mental illness, although difficult, painful, and sometimes humiliating and degrading, needn't lead to defeat. With hard work and empathic, passionate support, those who are suffering from mental illness can regain hope, build a sense of accomplishment, and survive.

What makes this book even more relevant and provocative is that most of the stories are written by therapists—mental health professionals including MSWs, PhDs, and MDs—many of whom have, themselves, confronted mental illness, just like the patients they are attempting to support and transform. *Same Time Next Week* demonstrates that knowledgeable, empathetic, and committed professionals can counter the institutional failure of which Dr. Kramer writes. But individual therapists can't make the changes necessary to reform a system that has been going in the wrong direction for decades—and perhaps longer. Our leaders in Washington and in local and state government must take steps to increase funding, expand facilities, and respond to the needs not only of patients but also of the professionals who are committed to helping them. And the public—that is, all of us—must do our part by acknowledging not only the struggle patients and families face but also their great potential to return to their jobs and their neighborhoods and to lead healthy and productive lives.

....

Lee Gutkind's book Stuck in Time: The Tragedy of Childhood Mental Illness *has recently been reissued by Open Road Integrated Media. He is Distinguished Writer in Residence at the Consortium for Science Policy and Outcomes at Arizona State University.*

ACKNOWLEDGMENTS
....

Same Time Next Week was made possible through support from the Jewish Healthcare Foundation, whose primary mission is to support healthcare services, education, and research, and to encourage medical advancement and protect vulnerable populations. On behalf of the Creative Nonfiction Foundation and the contributors to this collection, I would like to thank Karen Wolk Feinstein, Nancy Zionts, and their colleagues at the JHF for their vision and creativity as well as their ongoing encouragement and friendship.

Any book is the work of many people. I would like to thank, most of all, Landon Houle and Anne Horowitz for their editorial skill and invaluable dedication to the project; Jamie Beaudoin for her commitment and perseverance; Melissa Irr Harkes for legal vetting; Chelsea Denard, Katie McGrath, Matt Spindler, Shannon Swearingen, and Chad Vogler for fact checking and proofreading; Ken Thompson for his advice and counsel; the many writers who generously sent their work for consideration; and the entire staff at *Creative Nonfiction* and In Fact Books.

In addition, I am grateful to the Juliet Lea Hillman Simonds Foundation; the Consortium for Science, Policy, and Outcomes and the Hugh Downs School of Human Communication at Arizona State University; and the Pennsylvania Council on the Arts, all of whose ongoing support has been essential to the Creative Nonfiction Foundation's success.

Some names and identifying details have been changed to protect the identities of people and institutions mentioned in these essays.

BEYOND DESPAIR: THE GIFT OF RECOVERY

Karen Wolk Feinstein

O ccasionally, I see a movie I just can't forget. Something in it grabs me and won't let go. That's what happened after I saw *The Woodsman*, starring Kevin Bacon. It's the story of a pedophile who is released from prison and fights his way back to "normalcy," living painfully in a world that finds his obsession repugnant, but where temptation lurks in every public space.

Let me acknowledge that I have no therapeutic credentials whatsoever, that my musings are ill informed, and that my preoccupation with this story resulted from pure curiosity. I couldn't stop thinking about it; it seemed to lead to so many bigger questions about the way we treat mental illness in this country. There may be no "cure" for the more extreme psychological conditions, but is there something that can make life worth living, minimize the pain of a mental affliction, and allow some measure of daily joy and peace? What circumstances permit progress, ameliorate suffering, and offer restorative healing? *The Woodsman* is fictional, of course, but are there other, equally fascinating—and true—stories of people who have struggled with serious behavioral problems and achieved some triumph?

So I did what I often do when I'm inspired by such questions: I turned to Lee Gutkind, the mastermind of *Creative Nonfiction* and procurer of interesting and articulate stories about real life. My request was that he mobilize his usual connections among writers to unearth other journeys from dark to light. I had high expectations, but even so, I was dazzled by the hundreds of stories that poured forth—almost five hundred in all. I read the best submissions with keen interest and deliberation: what was there to be learned from these awesome struggles with mental demons? I wasn't expecting tales of miraculous cures, so I was prepared for the up and down nature of coping. And I was glad to see that although happy endings were not universal— some stories ended with suicide or less than optimal emotional health—every author documented significant progress, and some describe remarkable achievements. And the stories display rich insights and dramatic quests for sanity and equilibrium.

My own conclusions: some people benefit greatly from a good therapist; some, from finding the right medication; some, from a seemingly spontaneous improvement; some, from a combination of the above. What surprised me most were the common threads. Having a loving and responsive mother (or significant parental figure) seems to be preventive; having a loving and caring adult partner is restorative. Regardless, progress seldom comes in a straight line: courage, determination, and patience are required in large measure.

I hope that these stories elicit optimism about treating severe mental illness and help remove some of the stigma. With my interest in this topic having been sparked by a story about pedophilia, I realize that I was dealing with possibly the most feared and loathsome of conditions. However, Kevin Bacon's character in *The Woodsman* concludes his story by acknowledging that although his struggle not to harm young girls will probably never end, he *can* master his emotions, achieve a satisfying adult relationship, and work to restore the trust and confidence of others. I think that's a happy ending.

....

Karen Wolk Feinstein, PhD, is president and chief executive officer of the Jewish Healthcare Foundation (JHF) and its two supporting organizations, the Pittsburgh Regional Health Initiative (PRHI) and Health Careers Futures (HCF). Appointed as the Foundation's first president, Dr. Feinstein has become widely regarded as the national leader in healthcare quality improvement and often presents at national and international conferences. She is the author of numerous regional and national publications on quality and safety; she was the editor of the Urban & Social Change Review, *and she is the editor of the book* Moving Beyond Repair: Perfecting Health Care. *Additionally, she has served on the faculties of Boston College and Carnegie Mellon University, and taught at the University of Pittsburgh.*

PLAYING CARDS WITH MR. NEWMAN

J. Timothy Damiani

For long-term residents of a psychiatric ward, recovery is too often only a dim possibility. But, as a new psychiatrist discovers, sometimes reaching beyond one's own suffering and truly connecting with others (along with the right combination of meds) can work miracles.

Mental illness had wadded Mr. Newman into a ball, tossed him into a state hospital, and left him there as unceremoniously as one dumps a piece of trash. When I met him, he'd already been a patient for fifteen years.

As the new psychiatrist, I introduced myself to all thirty-eight patients on the all-male ward.

"Hi," I said again and again. "I'm Dr. Damiani."

Some of the men found my name a humorous tongue twister. *Dr. Donnie-ago? Dr. Dumb-ee-on-nee?* Others disparaged my profession, heritage, or both. "A wop shrink," they said. For a few, my presence as a young professional inspired sage advice. "Good to meet you, young fellow. You have your work cut out for you here."

But Mr. Newman didn't speak or move. At first, he didn't respond at all.

I leaned forward, not so close as to be within reach, but near enough to convey a sincere desire to communicate. "Some of the other patients have been calling me Dr. D."

Mr. Newman only tucked his head farther between his knees. With his arms around his legs, he squeezed himself tighter. His miserable withdrawal felt intensely private.

"I can come back later," I said, "if you don't want to talk now."

The unstructured routine of the state hospital seemed to stretch time. Life for chronic residents was one long sigh. There would be plenty of time to come back.

I was about to move on when Mr. Newman lifted his head just enough to peer over his legs. His face, bereft of emotion for years now, was eerily smooth. Thin and translucent, his skin was more like a plastic anatomy dummy's than a human's. He stared at an empty spot to my right and moaned, "I'm dead. The whole world is dead."

His fragile white arms, alarming in their delicateness, went to his head. With a hand over each ear, he moaned, "Dr. D. Dr. Death. We are all dead."

He rewrapped his legs, buried his face in his thighs, and rocked. Urine stains on his pants mapped the duration of his apathy. This withered patient and his unfettered hopelessness terrified me more than any of the others I had met. Mark Newman lived without being alive. He reminded me of my mother.

Mom was never a normal mom, and we were never a normal family. It was more accurate to say I lived in an orphanage where we all just happened to be related. Depression made my mother invisible. As a toddler, I routinely searched our house for her. One day, when I found her lying in bed, I climbed up over her knees. I wriggled next to her stomach, but after several minutes of fidgeting, she never moved. So I climbed away and went to play with my blocks.

Another time, after I'd just started school, I pulled her to the front door so she could watch me do bike tricks. Coasting with my feet between the handlebars, I glanced back. She smiled for a half second, then turned around and disappeared for the rest of my childhood. In my teenage years, after Dad officially left to be with another woman and her family, Mom sat in a chair in a corner of our house wearing a poncho, three sombreros, and dark sunglasses. This Mexican ghost of depression never spoke, rarely got up, and only nodded on occasion.

In the absence of parental guidance, I was raised by the television. *Rudolph the Red-Nosed Reindeer* gave me a vision of how to fit in, albeit as a misfit; *Charlie's Angels* proved big breasts had special power; *The Waltons* assured me love existed out there somewhere; and *American Bandstand* verified that every average American danced through a happy life.

A mother's love, by contrast, would have taught me how to express my love and accept being loved. But the prison of Mom's depression kept her affection from me and mine from her. I was never physically abused, and I was always fed. Mom was kind and gentle, and I sensed that she cared deeply for me. But we never acknowledged each other or managed to express any emotional connection. The only feeling I remember was a deep need to be noticed, to matter to someone—to anyone.

When I started school, I found affection elsewhere in whatever shape it took: extra attention from teachers, friendship with my peers, and care from their parents. Later, I discovered girls who shared my craving for acceptance and affection. By the end of high school, I had wrapped myself in a patchwork quilt of substitute love, but in the end, the rags and scraps weren't enough to provide any real comfort. What I thought was love had no real substance, no unifying force or fidelity.

Things began to change when I became a husband and a father. My wife and I bonded as we struggled to be good parents. I instantly loved my kids and they loved me. Their affection for me was genuine, and instinctively, I wanted the best for them. At our house, we entertained other families who had children of similar age. We set up play dates for the kids. I even learned to decorate a Christmas tree. Finally, I had a real family in which I belonged. Gradually the feelings of being unloved dissipated, and until I met Mr. Newman, I believed I'd moved beyond my painful past.

But the old ache in my throat returned when I saw Mark. I'd only stuck a Band-Aid over the wounds of my mother's depression, and Mark had ripped it away.

I had no idea how I would handle seeing him in this depressed state every day. Professionally I knew the odds of a positive outcome were small. Mark had been sick too long. No one would blame me if he didn't get better, no one except me. But despite all my fears and doubts, having a family to support was a kind of anchor. For their sakes, I couldn't just give up on Mark. I would do the best I could. After all, Mark wasn't my mother, and I was no longer the helpless son. My world was different now. I looked down at Mark and convinced myself things would be okay.

I went to the nursing station and read his story. I was searching for something to doctor. The chart said he suffered from schizophrenia but made little mention of profound depression. I phoned his sister for more information. My call surprised her. She and the rest of the family had lost contact with Mark, his mental illness erasing him from their lives. After her initial shock, she welcomed my questions about Mark and the chance to talk about what he was like before his illness. She described a flamboyant Romeo. Even allowing for a natural tendency to eulogize the past, the history she gave was far from that of a man with schizophrenia, and her memories made me wonder if he'd been misdiagnosed.

Most people suffering from schizophrenia don't engage with others. The illness tends to make them withdrawn, isolative, and socially clumsy. Mark had been a man of big appetites, several romances, and, for a period, he'd been a good father to his daughter. His past was more consistent with that of a man suffering from bipolar illness. He engaged with the world in periods of intense energy and then languished in apathetic depressions for long stretches, a melancholy that in Mark's case was also psychotic.

He received antipsychotic and antidepressant medications, but none helped. Given his history, I changed his prescription, combining lithium, a mood stabilizer, with a new antipsychotic agent.

Mark had been on the combination for three weeks when the staff and I noticed a small change. One day, he lifted his face from between his knees and focused on his fingers. Then he glanced around the room before resting his head back down. It wasn't much, but looking back, I see that he was engaging the world in tolerable bits, pairing the familiar with the new as his brain sparked to life.

Gradually, he began to eat more. He chewed faster and took larger bites. He eventually took the spoon from a surprised aide and shoveled the potatoes himself. Soon he took a bath without needing to be bribed, threatened, or coerced. For the first time in a long time, Mark began using the bathroom regularly instead of urinating on his pants or emptying himself in his chair.

As he left the restroom the staff would pound him on the back and lavish him with pun-filled praise:

"Way to go!"

"I always knew you had it in you."

Besides going about the necessities of a functioning life, what does a person waking up after fifteen years do with his time? After coming out of his tomb, our Lazarus played cards and told tales about buxom women. When it came to the ladies, rules were easy for Mark to recall, but not so for card games. We collected cards, and he threw them down haphazardly. At first, it was like trying to play with a two-year-old.

Then randomly some rules returned. Mark would be saving threes for gin, and then his brain would switch to crazy eights. He'd start matching the suit of my discard with his, ultimately confounding both of us. Or at other times, he would collect cards and never throw any away. One time, he threw a king on my queen and then took the whole pile as if we were playing war.

Growing up, I couldn't seem to do anything to earn my mother's affection, but I learned that others responded warmly when I performed well on the basketball court. As a result, I developed a competitive nature that distinguished me as an all-state basketball player. Mom predictably wasn't interested in my athletics. On the rare occasion I mentioned a victory, she would tell me I should have let the other boys win so they wouldn't feel bad. Then she'd sink back into a disappointed silence.

Only with Mark did I heed her advice. I wanted Mark to win at cards because it meant victory for both of us. He held his cards so loosely I could see his whole hand. I'd just match the rules of the day to his cards and then proclaim his success.

"Oh my goodness," I'd say, feigning surprise. "You have two fives, three eights, and four red cards. You won!"

Our games always ended with him laughing about pulling out a last-second conquest.

Mark was steadily improving, and the rules didn't remain jumbled for long. As time passed, the directives of crazy eights, war, old maid, and go fish all slowly came back.

"Dr. D.," he'd say. "I don't think two pairs work for four-of-a-kind. I think they all have to be the same number."

"You know, Mark," I'd say. "I vaguely remember something like that now that you mention it."

Shit, I'd think. *Now how will I let him win?*

After Mark began remembering the rules, many of our games ended in draws. Such interactions were fun but also served as real therapy for Mark.

Depression is sometimes called pseudo-dementia, as the apathy and cognitive deficits it produces mimic dementia. But Mark wasn't demented. He hadn't lost the machinery to make memories and plan ahead. These skills were just atrophied. He needed to exercise his brain and remember how to remember. In our games he was forced to access old memories while remembering his current cards. He needed to keep his hand upright, pay attention to my moves, plan ahead with his own schemes, and stay engaged in the present moment, all while other patients meandered by and offered their input. The concentration and effort were just what a rehabilitating brain needed.

Meanwhile Mark's libido grew at the same pace as his memory.

"Hey, Mrs. Jones," he called to a well-proportioned female staff member. "How about playing strip poker?"

"No, Mark," she said. "I don't think the hospital allows that."

"Come on," he teased. "I promise if you try it with me, you'll live forever." His face, fuller now and less translucent, beamed. Though he was joking, there was a sincere vigor to his plea. Sex—with its natural goal of reproduction—is quite the opposite of death and dying. I thought back to Mark calling me Dr. Death, and his statement about all of us being dead. Now he was telling the staff member how she could live forever. I took it as another sign of his healing.

As a result of Mark's resurrection, I gained a reputation as some kind of miracle medication guru. It felt good and bad. Mark had lost fifteen years of his life to a mental illness. He took some pills, and either the drugs or our attention and affection had returned him to health.

Whatever was the cause of Mark's recovery, what of my mom? How would our lives have changed if she had been successfully treated with medication? My dad, when he was around, never saw his way to bring her for treatment. Maybe he was ashamed or embarrassed. Or perhaps some bias of Mom's had prevented her from seeing a physician. By the time I was old enough to help, she refused our repeated efforts to take her to a doctor.

Mom was never actively suicidal or harmful to others, so forcing her into treatment would have been impossible. At times I wondered whether it *was* the attention that helped Mark get better, the same attention Mom refused. Was she always doomed?

The staff praised God for Mark's recovery. At the time, I was too conflicted to echo them. God and I had a long history, and these events came at a point of great confusion in my faith. When we moved to Florida, my family stopped attending church. But later as a teenager, I resurrected my Catholic faith and became a fervent practitioner. I prayed endlessly and believed wholeheartedly in God's providence for my life. I carried God into adulthood, though new questions arose, not the least of which was how could I reconcile a loving God who said humans had free will in a world beset with mental illness? I even spent a year working as a psychiatrist for a group of mentally ill priests, and despite my hopes, I never found the miraculous place where spirituality and mental illness could coexist.

To "credit" God with providing a cure for Mark didn't satisfy me. Would that mean God had permitted the illness to come to Mark? That He had let Mark's suffering go untreated for fifteen years before choosing to heal him? And what of Mom and her lack of any real recovery? Had God chosen *not* to heal her?

When it came to praising God for Mark's recovery, I couldn't. I kept choosing to ignore the glaring contradictions between faith in God, the concept of free will, and the stark reality of mental illness. It was simpler for me to tell myself that sometimes medications helped, sometimes they hurt, and sometimes they did nothing. Depression was a haphazard illness that stripped many people of their will to live. Mark's "cure" and Mom's stagnation were proof of that randomness, not evidence for God. I felt certain Mark's healing was not divine.

Still he got better and better, and he laughed more and more. Wrinkles formed on his aging cheeks. He was an odd sight, too old to be young and too young to be old. He spooked visiting children. They were bothered by not being able to discern his age, but he eventually charmed them. He would pick up the babies, hug them, and wink at the older children.

He told one woman that her son "was adorable and going to be a leader someday." He told another mother that her daughter had "so much life in her." By the time they left and he waved a silly good-bye to them, the children laughed at the weird, friendly man. Despite my internal doubts, my daily external experience of Mark felt spiritual. Seeing his urge to live inspired me, inspired all of us. How could he be so fragile and so resilient? There had never been a guarantee that he would come back from his illness. Lithium or a new medication or kindness could have failed. Mark could have given up, and who would ever blame him?

I didn't go to God, but I couldn't help but be drawn to Mark.

A couple of months passed. Most of the men on the ward had been chronically ill for years, and there were no other miracle cures. But the staff had an abundance of affection for the residents. I, too, began to find pleasure in their eccentric company. We were their family, whether they wanted us or not.

The relationships I formed with Mark, the other residents, and the staff were new to me. In my work life, I generally didn't rely on other people. I never asked for help, preferring to do the job myself. I always carried the burden of responsibility, and the constant weight kept me tense and distant from others. But working at the hospital, I began to relax. Despite being paid little, the staff was caring toward the residents. Many acted out of goodness, not for recompense. As I grew to trust them, I became less isolated. I was in a community where the burden could be shared. I began to have faith that we could all work together to help the residents. I decided to take a week off.

After my vacation, I returned to find Mark sullen. Gone was his hard-earned smile. The happy glint in his blue eyes had drained away. That first day back, he wouldn't talk to me. He stared into the distance, as if he were witnessing some trauma I couldn't see. I ordered some labs and waited. The second day, he finally spoke.

"I am a pool table," he said, "and I keep making the eight ball. No one wants to play with me."

I wasn't sure how I should respond. "Oh," was all I could muster.

"In the pool hall," he went on, "they call me a crazy fuck who keeps making the eight ball. I just gave blood."

"I know," I said, grateful for some information to which I could respond. "I ordered the test. I'm your doctor."

"If you are a doctor then you're not a pool table," Mark said.

What had happened to him? Maybe the improvement had all been imagined. Maybe I had caused his depression by leaving. Maybe Mark—like my mother—had swallowed too much of the darkness, and it was resurfacing with a renewed vengeance, killing him piece by piece.

He kept groaning, "I screwed up. I thought the world was small, but I've been alive for a hundred million years."

Lazarus headed back into the grave. Had I gotten too close, pushed him too hard, gone too fast? Even a positive stress is stress on a weakened brain.

"I'm dead," he moaned. More than any phrase, this one devastated me.

"What's being dead feel like?" I asked.

"Being dead is nothing," Mark said. "I'll be dead forever."

"I feel that way sometimes too." My response seemed comical in comparison to his misery, and yet I did know the nothingness of not feeling loved by my mother, the nothingness of no one noticing I existed.

"You don't want to be dead," Mark said. "The staff made me take a bath."

"You do smell good." Soap, in my mind, was akin to cleanliness, which in turn suggested the health that I so badly wanted for Mark.

"What's the hell in smelling good?" Mark said. A dirt stain circled his neck. His wrongly buttoned shirt flared out in misalignment. "I'm dead," he went on. "If I'm dead, you're dead. What do you want to be dead for?"

I had no answers. A bitter part of me felt fooled. I should have known depression always won. There was no caring God with cures up his sleeve. There were only delusions, and Mark's cure was the biggest mirage of all. In that moment, I felt as though there was no reason to keep trying, to keep kicking against the wall of mental illness and the inevitability of our doomed futures.

The blood work indicated Mark's lithium level was low. Uninspired, I raised the dose, watched, and waited. My sorrow deepened. I missed Mark and our card games. I missed the hope his life evoked.

In those first days I negotiated with my bitter side. Mark had at least been well for a little while. Maybe I ought to be thankful for even a small recovery rather than demand he stay better. Was there a minimum time requirement for a healing to matter? We get colds and heart attacks and cancers again and again. Mark had relapsed but he'd had a few good days. Couldn't I be okay with that? Wasn't even one day unburdened by the despair of depression worth something?

The return of his depression forced me to consider other more meaty questions of life. Could I live with the inevitability of pain and mental illness? Could I still work for healing knowing it was fickle?

After about seven days on the increased dose of lithium Mark moaned to me, "You are a millionaire from New York."

"I wish," I said.

But compared to him I *did* feel like a millionaire. I had a healthy family and a mind capable of joy. I felt guilty for my riches, but also thankful. And from within that gratitude, I sensed I had begun to change. My anger about my past had genuinely decreased. I had learned to let the sadness meet the air of grief and thus begin to heal. I could sit with Mark and accept his fate. He might never get better.

As if hearing my thoughts Mark said, "Do I smell good? Smelling good means you're dead. Why do you want me dead?"

"I don't want you dead," I answered.

Mark paused, then asked, "Are you alive?"

I told him I was.

"If you are alive," he said, "then I am alive. But I'm not alive."

Again, I didn't know what to say, so I said nothing.

Mark patted me on the back. "You're a nice guy," he said.

I didn't want to be nice. I didn't think niceness fit in a world where depression damaged so many for so long.

I waited and counted the days after the lithium change.

Day 1:

"You look good, Mark."

"I don't feel good."

"You want to play cards?"

"If we play cards, the whole world will blow up."

Day 2:

"I'm dead. I'm not supposed to be alive. I've got no father and no mother. Dr. D., go home with your family. Engineer Jesus, let Dr. D. go home with his family. Don't stay here. You're not here. It's osmosis. You aren't really here."

Day 3:

"Hey, Mark, let's go to the patio."

"Don't make me go to the patio."

"I won't make you, but it might be fun."

"No," he said, but sat up on his bed to talk. "How's the family?" he asked.

Day 4:

"Mark, you ever think of going to a place near your sister?"

"My family is dead. I'm the only one alive. Maybe I'll go to Florida. I heard it's nice there."

"You said you are alive," I said. "Do you want to be alive?"

"I guess so. I haven't got a choice."

"You could wish you were dead. Some people even want to commit suicide. Do you ever think of suicide?"

"No," Mark said. "I want to be alive."

Day 5:

"Dr. D., you want to play cards?"

"Yes," I said.

I wanted to play cards more than Mark could ever imagine.

The game went well. His knowledge of the rules hadn't been erased by his relapse. I threw a five down, knowing he had been saving them. Instead of taking it and building a winning hand, he reached to draw from the stack. I didn't have the heart to correct his mistake. I decided to wait for another way to make his victory look more accidental. He put the new card in his hand and threw a three onto the discard pile. I was saving threes, and if Mark was his old self, he would have known that. In fact, if I took the three, I would win. I reached for the deck instead.

He stopped my hand in mid-reach. "Weren't you saving threes?"

I stuttered. "Yeah," I finally said, following his gaze to the discard pile. I tried to play it off. "How did I miss that?" I said. "I'm glad we aren't playing for money."

I locked eyes with him. A shiver shot through me. I understood then that Mark had purposely not picked up the five I'd thrown down, which in all probability would have given him the victory. Mark had been waiting to find a way for me to win.

Out from underneath the imprisonment of his depression peeked Mark, a good man who wanted me to feel better. He'd been enslaved by his moods and abused by his neurochemicals. He had lost most of what I would claim as meaningful, and yet he was looking after me. He offered me some small consolation as we traversed the shared inescapable misery life sometimes gives. Here was a simple act of inexpressible kindness, a generosity that neutralized depression's hopelessness. It represented a part of Mark that mental illness could not take away.

"In fact"—I picked up the card—"that is exactly what I need." I slapped my winning hand onto the table. I claimed everything: the victory, the mystery, the pain, the confusion, the uncomfortable favoritism, the fickleness, the tragedy, and the doubts.

Mark laughed and smiled, and in that moment, his face was enough. I didn't need answers.

Gratefully, Mark never sunk back into his psychotic depression again. The stability of his mood and the clarity of his thinking stuttered forward in rusty lurches, but the overall trend kept him moving in the direction of health. After several months he reached a point where we could relax. Soon he was discharged to a facility near his family.

I was thankful to have known Mark. He was proof that even when mental illness stretches into years, recovery is still possible. If I'm worried about a patient relapsing, I remember Mark's course and find some comfort.

But when I think of Mark now, it isn't his exceptional recovery I remember most. Rather, I am filled with an abiding appreciation of the significant roles we played in each other's lives. We both faced certain challenges. Yet, in the middle of our struggles, we built a meaningful relationship. We helped one another. Maybe this is how God works.

The best my reason can do is to acknowledge that something extraordinary occurred. One hand of cards began a deeper transformation in me. I grew in my ability to tolerate despair, and I learned to listen to the raw voice of suffering without running away. With Mark, I began to feel a sense of connection and confidence that has helped me sit patiently in the dark corners of hospitals with so many other troubled people and not lose hope.

....

J. Timothy Damiani has published academic articles in medical journals, and his nonfiction work has appeared in RiverLit, r.kv.r.y, *the* Gainesville Sun, *and the anthology* Flashlight Memories. *As a practicing psychiatrist and father, he has spent the last twenty years learning about life from his children, as well as from his elderly male patients at a state hospital.*

HOPE NURTURES THE DREAM

Ronald Bassman

A young man with dreams of becoming a psychologist finds himself in the midst of his own mental health crisis. Will an official diagnosis stand in the way of his ambitions, or can he learn to use his personal experience to inspire others?

In February of 2014 I gave testimony opposing a bill that was quickly moving through the Vermont legislature. The bill, which would allow the forced administration of psychiatric drugs to outpatients on a nonemergency basis, was intended to improve the quality of services and save money. As an invited expert I cited research and personal experience to demonstrate that the stated purpose for the bill would not be accomplished. While psychiatric drugs can stabilize people in the short term, I pointed out, their use leads to physical problems, many of which are irreversible. Moreover, when patients are not given a choice in their treatment, their spirits are broken, and the driving forces of recovery—hope and possibility—are severely diminished. For too long the coerced stabilization of those who look, feel, think, and act differently was thought to be the sole possibility. My journey, along with those of an increasing number of my peers, exposes this to be a myth.

. . .

Like far too many others, during my transition from adolescent to adult I was forced to abandon youthful hopes and dreams and become forever identified as a mental patient. Less than a year after earning a master's degree in psychology, I was hospitalized and spent my twenty-third birthday confined to the seclusion room of a psychiatric hospital. My parents, upon seeing their once-promising son thinking and behaving so differently, were driven to attempt just about any intervention to bring me back into the fold, so little did they know of what awaited me once I was committed to the hospital and labeled (diagnosed) schizophrenic.

From behind the locked seclusion room door, I shouted until I was hoarse. "You can't do this to me. I did nothing wrong. I have rights. This is not fair. I'll sue . . . I'll get all of you." Comedian George Carlin declared in one of his classic riffs, "Rights aren't rights if someone can take them away. They're privileges."

I learned firsthand about my rights when my cries were answered by two burly psychiatric aides and a nurse. Stripped of my clothes and held down, I was given a not-very-gentle injection to my butt. This daily confrontation was re-enacted again and again and culminated repeatedly in my being tied in restraints. It was only when my spirit was broken and I learned to accept their demands for absolute compliance that I was given a small number of hospital privileges—for example, the freedom to pace the hall in a futile attempt to decrease the deadening effects of the psychiatric drugs.

Crazy. Many people have asked me what it was like. How did it start? Was I really mad? No one recovers from schizophrenia, they say, were you misdiagnosed? I try to explain that the term *madness* is generic. My experiences and those of fellow travelers may have similar elements, but in their complex wholes they are different and defy all of the falsely uniform diagnoses and one-way formulaic treatments.

At twenty-two, I was not the person I wanted to be. I did not like or respect myself. My first episode started when I perceived madness to be my path to transformation. I believed that I would be able to abandon my unwanted timid identity, reject consensual reality, and immerse myself in the mad world of unlimited possibilities. In the beginning, I did not feel threatened. There was much to be enjoyed and relished in my new specialness. I had the power to see and hear what others did not. I could exert control over television programs and create new and better endings for films. Television news commentators spoke in code with secret messages that were just for me. Divisions within our country over the Vietnam War signaled to me that those in authority were spreading propaganda and misinformation. I believed I was being called to bring about peace. Boredom was vanquished by all of the moment-to-moment discoveries. I predicted the future and when people challenged me and tried to point out my errors, I refused to change my beliefs.

A few childhood friends tried to understand but were confused by my uncharacteristic behavior. They had never been privy to the part of me that had always tried to hide fears that badgered the otherwise bright and sensitive youngster I'd appeared to be. Or maybe they did know. Despite my efforts they must have seen my hands shake when I lit a cigarette or when I played billiards. I was not built to be the cool fearless hero of the then-popular cowboy movies. Saturated with my unhappiness, feeling disconnected from everyone, I chose to be different, to explore an alternate path. I leaped into the abyss of madness, and instead of hiding who I was, I became, "look at me and what I can do."

But once you reject consensual reality, once you step across the line into forbidden territory, once choice becomes compulsion, you may not be able to return. Letting go of inhibition, I was attracted to the bright light without understanding that the dark must also be acknowledged. The yin and yang of life, the soft and the hard, was wisdom I had not yet learned. I was fascinated by Zen and Taoist paths to enlightenment states, but my innocence, my lack of training and knowledge about alternative realities, made all explanations equally plausible. I did not know that in the practice of Zen meditation what I was experiencing would be called *makyo*, the illusions or hallucinations that come as one progresses in meditation practice toward enlightenment.

Soon my early hopes changed into intense fears that bordered on panic. I felt the terror of being alone, of being an outsider who was unable to communicate, who was afraid of everyone and everything. I sensed the presence of dark inexplicable forces. I knew with certainty that I must be on guard and exquisitely sensitive to danger. Trust no one. They will try to trick you. Of one thing I was sure: the fate of the world depended upon me and what I did.

I stumbled down false trails and into exaggerated notions of self-importance. Familiar feelings of insecurity and powerlessness, oxygenated with mistrust and skepticism, set loose a pervasive fear that I had never before felt. Paranoia is the name the mental health experts give to that constellation of thoughts and feelings. The fears kept increasing as if they would continue to get stronger until my mind exploded like a flimsy balloon. Existing in a waking nightmare, I could not shake the feeling that I had inadequate protection from the eyes of strangers. I had little capacity to erect a barrier that would shield my mind from their invasive probing. A constant malignant presence was out there, waiting to subdue and enslave me. My world was becoming increasingly unpredictable. Every sound and smell had to be attended to and judged as a potential trick or trap. The universe was engaged in a war between good and evil, and unless I fulfilled my mission to convert people to goodness, a severe disaster would occur. I was partially right: there was a war going on, but it was a struggle within myself. My inability to find a way to integrate the warring identity conflicts within me made me the first casualty of a private battle that would soon be made public.

I had blindly jumped into the sea of madness without knowing its depth and without forethought of whether I would be able to master the roiling waters. But the most profound danger, as I was soon to discover, would come from the psychiatric interventions used to force me back into the reality I had rejected. Like a deep-sea diver pulled too quickly from the depths without the necessary slow decompression, I became helplessly disorientated. My life trajectory was forcibly propelled onto a new course by my so-called rescuers. Mental health professionals, led by psychiatrists, are given a mandate to bring back those who have wandered off the well-trod, acceptable path. My unwillingness to give up being in control of my journey became a battle of wills. A fierce survival battle for me but not to the hospital staff, who saw me as just another unruly patient who would eventually understand who held the power. I naively thought that if they weren't able to break my resolve they would have to release me.

Four months into my first hospital stay, I still managed to resist and refuse to assure my psychiatric helpers that I would strive to return to what they called my premorbid condition. I did not want to let go of my newfound spirit and return to hiding in the self-constrained persona I had abandoned. The massive doses of Thorazine and Stelazine they forced upon me did not subdue me to their satisfaction. I struggled to hold on to my new identity. I believed that submission to their demands would crush my soul.

The hospital psychiatrists decided to bring on their most powerful and dangerous intervention. They prescribed a treatment course of forty insulin comas combined with electroshock. I was unable to resist the mind-bending effects of the comas. Each coma would last for up to an hour, and patients would be revived by the intravenous administration of glucose. Memory loss was common, and the treatments occasionally resulted in death. I have often wondered what theory or explanation could possibly provide a rationale for putting a person in a coma—or, for that matter, for administering any of the other dangerous and invasive treatments that infamously mark the history of psychiatry. Perhaps a clue can be found in the writing of acclaimed New Zealand author Janet Frame: "'For your own good' is a persuasive argument that will eventually make a man agree to his own destruction."

All of the young men and women who became unwilling members of the insulin coma group were chosen because we were the treatment-resistant, rebellious, noncompliant irritants who were not sufficiently responsive to the psychiatric drugs. Insulin coma therapy, intended to shock the patient into "reality," is a sledgehammer blow to the brain that breaks the spirit. Our minds were treated like the old cathode ray tube televisions: when the picture got fuzzy, you shook or kicked the console. Sometimes it worked better for a while and sometimes the TV was damaged beyond repair. Less than two years after my hospital sojourn, insulin treatments were largely relegated to the notorious category of invasive somatic treatments that are no longer used for treatment.

Our treatment sessions occurred five days a week for eight weeks. Every morning before breakfast we were marched into the gray surreal basement of the hospital. Each of us, confined to our respective beds, would be injected with enough insulin to put us into a coma. When we lost consciousness, our hands and feet were bound to prevent injury from seizures. The medical staff considered their purposeful destruction of our brain cells far more acceptable than an accidentally broken bone during a treatment convulsion. My insistence on the validity of altered states of consciousness proved to them that I was mad. My treating doctor believed that putting patients into brain-damaging comas was healing. He was paid well for his brand of psychiatric madness.

I've forgotten much of what happened, but I can recall the terror flooding over me as I was forced to wake. Starting to rouse, I squirmed in the sweat-soaked sheets and tugged at the restraints as I searched for something familiar to ease the panic. Immobile, awake in a nightmare, I could not grasp who I was. I had lost my identity and all connections to time and place. A figure stood over me pressing a straw between my lips. A sweet wetness filled my mouth. Force-fed a sugar solution from a huge, seemingly bottomless container, I felt like I was drowning in the liquid I was drinking. I tried to understand what I was being told. The words became louder: "Swallow . . . drink up." It was as if I were being pulled from my grave while gagging on fluid that was being poured down my throat. The presence of death felt as real as the voice pressing me to drink the glucose back into my blood stream. I was falling into a black hole and, at the same time, I could feel someone pulling me back up and pouring and pouring and pouring liquid into me. With absolute certainty I knew that if I didn't do something, if I did not fight, I would die. But for which side should I fight? I did not know whether life was drinking and awakening, or letting myself fall to the bottom of the hole.

I fought to free myself from the straps around my ankles and wrists, but the only rewards for my efforts were the bruises whose origins I would later try to remember. I fought with all of my strength. My observers saw no fierce battle, merely the easily managed thrashings of an unruly child. A struggle representing a lifetime of tortuous indecision, of wavering between the poles of cooperation and rebellion, passivity and assertion, acceptance and challenge, was unworthy of anyone's attention. The unalterable fact was that I would be untied only when the liquid in the container had been drained. The war was waged only in my mind. The outcome had already been determined and always mocked me in the same way.

Upon finally reaching full consciousness, I passively waited for the rest of the group to be untied. Next, we were herded into the showers for our second rude awakening. Modesty ignored, we were blasted awake under the watchful eyes of psychiatric aides.

After eight weeks, the psychiatrist saw evidence of what he considered to be a successful treatment outcome: my absolute compliance. I agreed to his recommendations and answered his questions obediently, albeit very slowly. The insulin treatments had reached critical mass for spirit breaking. My senses were dulled and much of my memory was inaccessible to me. The medical staff were impressed with my progress. I became a good hospital patient and acquired privileges. Docile and trustworthy, I was moved to an unlocked room and after five months, I was permitted visitors. Less than a month later I was discharged.

Not far from Manhattan, on the New Jersey side of the Hudson River, there's a clearing among the trees and rocks where Alexander Hamilton fought his fatal duel with Aaron Burr. Before I became a mental patient I went there with friends to innocently laugh, play, and enjoy the self-centered exuberance of our youth. On those rocks, gazing across the river at the New York skyline, I first felt the charge of energy and power that would later tantalize and haunt me and evade my attempts to understand and control it.

After being discharged from my first hospital confinement I visited that spot. Sitting on those once-familiar rocks and staring off into the distance, I searched and waited for a feeling or memory to infuse my apathetic body with that mystical power the hospital staff had shocked out of me. Both in daylight and at night the results were the same. There was no magic to be recaptured. No opening of the mind and senses, just the dull pain of longing for what once was. Along with so many others praying and worshiping at their public and private shrines, I had joined the community of the disappointed and resigned.

My hospital discharge was contingent upon me seeing a psychotherapist. I asked this therapist, "How would I know if I was beginning to become psychotic again?"

Her response haunted me for years: "When you're feeling exuberant, really good, that's your warning sign." What did she mean by "really good"? How good was too good? She never explained this to me, and I wondered if I had to protect myself by living a life of unexciting blandness.

I continued with therapy and after three years passed, parts of my memory returned. Gradually, I began to think more clearly. I was working full time and I had begun applying to doctoral psychology programs. Since high school I had dreamed of becoming a psychologist. Now, I hoped that what I would learn in becoming a psychologist would protect me from being hospitalized again.

Unexpectedly, and shocking to everyone, when I was fairly sure that I was free of the specter of madness, I was hospitalized again. Just when I was feeling good about myself, confident that I was back on course, that I would become a psychologist and help others, I was back in a locked ward. I was devastated. I hated thinking that my therapist's admonition had been correct. Had I begun to feel too confident, too good? Was her dictum right, or was it just a seed that she'd planted? I did not want to believe that I could survive only if I existed in a narrow range of emotions. It took a long time before I could fully trash that too-blithe admonition.

After seven months I was discharged from my second psychiatric hospitalization and moved back into my parents' three-bedroom apartment in Newark, New Jersey. I again began the project of reconstructing myself. Fortunately, this state hospital had not administered any kind of shock treatment. Still, bludgeoned by heavy-duty psychiatric drugs, disheartened and depressed, I wondered if I had the will to attempt the Sisyphean task of recovery.

Despair and loneliness were my constant companions. I needed people. I wanted to be around people. But how do you relate when your feelings are dominated by fear and embarrassment? Emptiness, nothing to say, nothing to contribute. Only with anonymity as a shield could I be with people and not have to face my humiliating inadequacies.

My one relief was taking the brief bus ride from Newark to Manhattan. I found some solace in walking the streets of New York City. The walking mirrored the relentless pacing I had done in the hospital corridors; it seemed to be the one aspect of my life where I could claim some degree of control. How well I remember believing, in the months after my release from my second hospitalization, that a bleak future with no friends was my destiny. Marriage and children would not be available to one such as I. Dull and slow, devoid of spontaneity, I hardly had the energy to hate my life.

I, like most who have been diagnosed with schizophrenia, have been told that I have a biochemical disorder, a brain disease. To remain stable and survive outside of an institution, we are told, we must take psychiatric drugs for the rest of our lives. If we work, it has to be in low-pressure jobs with few demands. Quietly, almost inaudible even to myself, I said no. No, a psychologist I will become. I will not let go of my dream.

One year after that second discharge I was able to stop taking all psychiatric drugs and have remained drug-free for the past forty-plus years. Two years later, having been able to keep alive a spark of spirit, I found myself capable of completing a psychology internship in a psychiatric hospital and was then accepted into a doctoral psychology program. I did not reveal my hospitalizations to anyone at the university. In my studies, I found my personal experience an asset in understanding what is helpful and harmful to those struggling with disturbing and painful emotions. I knew of the importance of maintaining hope and the necessity of supportive relationships. Thus began my lifetime devotion to working with and advocating for people and families who have rejected the limitations of the mainstream treatments that deny one's capacity to fully recover.

The support of my family and friends and my stubborn resistance to the idea that I would always have to take psychiatric drugs fueled my recovery. I became aware that my personal experience could serve as an example of possibility for others. Perhaps most significant to my recovery was falling in love, getting married, and the birth of a son. Founded on trust, respect, and openness, our fully committed relationship was a source of growth and stability for both of us. The support of my little family enabled me to use what I had learned the value of compassion and empathy—in my work as a psychologist and my role as a husband and father.

I stood in the lobby of the Waldorf Astoria imagining how that magical name has long signified the intimidating entitlement of those with wealth and privilege. The old feeling of not belonging was a tiny hitchhiker traveling in my jacket pocket, reminding me of past discomfort and awkwardness. The stately, oh-so-proper elegance spoke of the pleasures of the winners. As I played with the irony, I felt my excitement grow. I was an invited speaker for the American Psychological Association's annual conference. The symposium was entitled *Empowering Psychologists Engaged in Public Service.*

Seeing me seated with the other speakers, the chairman greeted me and reminded me to stay within the twenty-minute time limit. He seemed even more anxious than I was when he told me that I would be the last of the four speakers. My new openness about my psychiatric history made me automatically wary of people's reactions. I thought of how much I had already cut from my presentation. Trying to speak for the misunderstood and oppressed who are historically lacking in voice does not accommodate well to brevity, nor to the objective distance elected to be worn by most mental health professionals.

Days of listening to other speakers redeveloping the same old club-driven issues fed my impatience. When my name was called, I took my place at the podium. At long last I had a credible voice and a forum. Ashamed no more, and no longer needing to hide my past schizophrenia label, I was here to help psychologists better understand the elements that contribute to genuine recovery. I spoke of what was helpful and what was harmful with the intent to inspire them to re-examine the myths hindering the development of new theories and services that promote recovery.

My talk at APA went well, but compliments and requests for reprints did not signify changes in establishment thinking about mental illness. I realized that their feelings of compassion and moral indignation would too quickly retreat and integrate with other information stored in the intellectual realm. The brief glimpse of drama seldom stirs the playgoer to meaningful actions. It was for me the beginning of a long career dedicated to expanding the rights, choices, and treatments of people struggling with serious mental illness. I firmly believe that there exists for each person the possibility of overcoming the travails of mental illness.

My wife, Lindsey, our six-year-old son, Jesse, and I walked up Broadway to find a restaurant. My presentation done, I savored the relief and allowed myself to feel the tiredness. A free-associating heightened awareness and a quiet joyfulness accompanied the fatigue.

More than twenty years had passed since I'd last visited the site of the Hamilton-Burr duel. My boyhood experience there now lingered as a fond memory rather than an active symbol of lost abilities. To our mutual surprise, Lindsey and I discovered in a meandering conversation that she too had memories of visiting that obscure historical site. We had already planned to have Jesse visit my brother in New Jersey after the conference, so we decided to see what that historic site elicited in us after so many years. The anticipated visit left me feeling a bit of apprehension. I wanted to go back there, but I also didn't. What if I did feel something extraordinary, would it upset my prized current stability?

Driving there, I realized that I had only a vague memory of where it was. We aimlessly drove around, almost like it was a test, like if it really mattered, fate or subconscious memory would guide me. I saw nothing familiar and, being pressed for time, I asked a policeman for directions. When we came to that once-familiar view of the New York City skyline, it seemed different. We searched for that remembered clearing among the wild growth but found only a small park with a neat lawn and wooden benches that could have been any one of the thousands of scenic overlooks that dot our country's highways. I gave up and started driving away when Lindsey noticed a small stone pillar with a bronze bust of Hamilton on top. Behind the pillar was a boulder whose engraving identified it as the place where Hamilton's head had rested after he was fatally wounded in the duel with Burr. Our mouths dropped open and our heads shook in unison, almost as if our disappointment were choreographed. The pillar seemed to us an arrogant attempt to transform a vibrant historic space, once a secret place of power, into a lifeless landmark.

I was angry, cheated of my test. How would I ever know the truth about that feeling of power and whether I could now handle it? The flash of feelings passed quickly and settled into a bemused recognition that I was childishly pouting over a not-so-important injustice. More importantly I was grateful to that place for the memories, dreams, and promises that had given me a measure of sustenance and strength during my most trying times.

Whether I had changed or the space had changed, I was okay. I had no wish to engage in a futile struggle to hold on to a myth of permanence. I felt strong in that moment, and thought that as long as I could search for and occasionally find parts of answers that generated more questions, I could live and die without clinging to some false certainty that I know the *absolute truth*.

Now, when I teach, the questions I am asked often center around my recovery, or what I prefer to call my transformation. How did I overcome the damning diagnoses—first schizophrenia, paranoid type, and, when hospitalized again, schizophrenia, chronic type? The word *chronic* conjures up images of the ubiquitous disheveled homeless person engaged in emotional dialogues with friends or adversaries that no one else can hear or see.

In order to get into a doctoral program and eventually become a licensed psychologist, I had to keep my past secret. Now, decades of being open brings to me precious freedom from shame and embarrassment, but it too has complications. In my current psychotherapy practice I have to decide whether disclosure would be genuinely helpful to the person who has come to see me. I question whether it would it put our relationship into a tight little box, skewing perceptions and becoming more of a distraction than a benefit. With the publishing of my writings my name turns up prominently in Google searches. Words like *schizophrenia, madness,* and *recovery* appear alongside my name for any prospective therapy client to see. My decision to be open precludes privacy in this electronic age. The positive: I am free to be me without reservation—nothing to hide. No threat of closeted secrets unexpectedly being exposed. I don't care if people know that I was locked up twice in psychiatric institutions. I know who I am and I am proud of my lifelong journey of growth and discovery.

After I became a psychologist I used my experience with madness to connect to those who also had lost the freedom to pursue their self-directed goals. I met peers with similar experiences fighting for changes in a mental illness treatment system that does not work. I learned that those of us who were forced into unwanted interventions and who refused to be submissive were treated the most harshly. Yet those few of us who survived and later thrived became the strongest activists. We were dedicated to making recovery a real possibility for anyone who struggled with their own unique form of madness. I became part of an emerging community of peers who fight for social justice.

In 2004 I was honored to receive the Ed Roberts Humanitarian Award from the Independent Living Center for People with Disabilities. When I was called to the dais to speak, I looked out at what seemed to me a family of kindred spirits, and saw much more than people with mental and physical challenges. I saw a diverse mix of individuals with unique strengths and weaknesses who fight every day to overcome emotional and physical barriers, along with prejudice and discrimination.

My acceptance speech leaned heavily on one of my mantras— the power of *hope* and *possibility*. I spoke of equal opportunity, fairness, and the fight for social justice. I said that most of the strong advocates I know can recall a particularly horrendous time during their treatment when they vowed to make sure that those who followed them would not face the same obstacles they had encountered. We would promote and fight for expanding the opportunity of each person, regardless of disability, to lead a life of quality and choices. We survived because we fought and refused to accept the dire prognoses and negative predictions heaped upon us. I am grateful for being able to do work that demands openness and encourages me to learn and keep growing. The challenges I faced gave me the opportunity to develop awareness and sensitivity. I ended my acceptance speech with my other mantra: *Never give up.*

During a recent discussion with my wife I thought of a conundrum. I am a strong advocate against the overuse and harmfulness of psychiatric drugs. Research has shown that these drugs do physical damage and inhibit recovery. So I wonder, what if a new drug is created that causes no harm and eliminates both wanted and unwanted symptoms? Would I favor the forced use of that drug? My answer is no. I believe that forcing people into treatments that they are opposed to hinders their potential for positive development.

The unresolved question: How can the needs of the community and the individual's desire to maintain his or her freedom be mediated in the dynamically changing environment in which we all live? I hope that we will be open to searching for new answers.

....

Ronald Bassman, diagnosed with schizophrenia in his early twenties, defied dire predictions to fully recover and become a licensed psychologist. He is the current chair of The Community Consortium, an organization that promotes the civil and human rights of people with psychiatric disabilities. A cofounder, with other ex-patients and allies, of the International Network Towards Alternatives for Recovery (INTAR), he has been an elected member of the American Psychological Association's Expert Taskforce on Serious Mental Illness and has served two terms as president of the National Association for Rights Protection and Advocacy (NARPA).

INSIDE

Dan Tomasulo

A therapist building his practice agrees to counsel a young woman intent on self-destruction. But when her troublesome behavior triggers memories of a painful loss, he threatens to end their sessions.

Something smelled wrong. A strange odor had begun seeping through the vent in my office. It was hard to identify: Bad meat? A dead animal? A poisonous chemical? My secretary, Dolores, was walking down the hall from the waiting room, covering her nose and mouth with her right hand, and holding a single sheet of paper, the initial interview sheet for my new patient, in the other. Dolores walked into my office and closed the door behind her. Rolling her eyes, she shook the paper in front of me and removed her hand from her mouth. She exhaled with a sigh, then inhaled through her nose and closed her eyes.

"This is a new low, even for you," she said.

"What do you mean?" I asked.

"Do you know anything about this girl?"

"Not really. Her physician said he had finally convinced her to come to therapy, and that she made a botched suicide from an overdose of Midol months earlier, and I agreed with him that no one seriously tries to do themselves in with Midol."

"Well, she is a piece of work. We are going to have to have the entire office sprayed after she leaves. She is filthy."

"She isn't homeless, is she?" I asked.

"She wrote down an address, but I doubt she lives with anybody—she seems too disgusting. Her hair is matted and she is dressed in rags, she smells, and she has tattoos all over her," Dolores said. "If you take her, I'm not coming in the days she is here. I won't be able to walk into a store afterwards!"

"Okay, take it easy. What kind of tattoos?"

"Homemade."

"She doesn't sound well. Do you want to show her in?"

"I don't think you want her down here on the leather chairs."

"Why not?"

"I am sure she has bugs."

"Bugs!"

"Yes, bugs. She stinks, has ugly infected homemade tattoos, wears clothes you couldn't give away, and has bugs crawling on her."

"I'll go down and meet her. What's her name?"

"Suzanne, but it says here on her information sheet she prefers to be called by her nickname."

"What's her nickname?"

"Cutter."

I asked Dolores not to follow me back to the waiting room, but to wait in the group room until I spoke to the new patient. I had a feeling that an extra person in the waiting room might make things uncomfortable, particularly if I had to talk to Suzanne on the spot.

When I had been a staff psychologist at a hospital, I saw who came in, did my assessment and treatment plan, and then got paid whether they ever showed up again or not. I was on my own now, still building my private practice as a psychologist. In New Jersey, you are supervised for 3,500 hours after completing your doctorate; then you take a written state exam, present a case study, take an oral exam, and wait six months to find out if you passed. Between the educational and supervisory requirements, you learn about testing, theory, transference, and countertransference, as well as how to make a referral, terminate a client, set a sliding scale, advertise ethically, refer for medicine, run groups, work with couples, deal with defiant children, manage dysfunctional families, and calm the flagrantly psychotic. To build a private practice I learned to do all of this.

But no one taught me how to deal with a smelly referral.

Suzanne was sprawled out on the couch, thumbing through a women's magazine. Her smell ambushed me as I walked toward her. It was all I could do not to vomit. This wasn't something that I could ignore or be aloof about. This was a serious stink, and I found myself involuntarily wincing and making faces as I approached her. At first glance she looked like a bad impersonation of Janis Joplin. She wore layers of clothes—more like layers of rags—and her dark brown hair was matted in some parts, but was mostly just dirty and stringy. High-top sneakers completed the costume.

On the back of her left hand was a homemade tattoo of an anchor. It was a drawing you would have expected from a three-year-old, but this was a nasty purple defacement on the hand of a nineteen-year-old.

"Hi, I'm Dan," I said.

She looked up at me, then went back to her magazine.

"Right," she said.

"I have a bit of a problem," I began.

"Great, a shrink who is telling me he has a problem," she said, and kept staring at the magazine.

"Actually, the problem is your hygiene. I would really like to talk with you, but it is too difficult for me to concentrate on anything else. I think you need to clean yourself up a bit before we can meet."

I couldn't believe the words coming out of my mouth. This seemed so unlike me, but I felt I had no choice.

"Aren't you people supposed to accept everyone?" she said with contempt in her voice.

"I only accept people to work with whom I feel I can help. I can't work with you until you do something about your body odor, I'm sorry."

"Hey, that's cool. I didn't really want to do this anyway," she said as she stood up.

"I will try to find you a clinic or a local hospital that might be willing," I told her. "I see on your information sheet that you've lived all your life here in New Jersey and that you currently live right here in Red Bank. Should I try to find a clinic or hospital that will take you near your home?"

"What for?" she said as she threw the magazine back on the table. "You guys can't really help me. This is all a bunch of crap anyway isn't it?"

"Maybe I should put that on the door," I said, as I started to laugh. "Dan Tomasulo, crap-ologist."

This also wasn't like me. I don't typically make jokes with patients I am meeting for the first time.

"Maybe it's *me* who doesn't want to see *you*!" she said. "Oh, I'm sorry, I'd *really* like to talk with you, but you'd have to get rid of these stupid paintings and stop making lame jokes. Then maybe we could meet, but don't get your hopes up; I'll just find something else wrong with you."

She was bright and spirited, and despite the intense attempt to make herself repulsive, there was an innocence and spark underneath it all. I offered an option.

"Good point," I said. "How about a plan B: Why don't we start today by doing our session outside? We can walk and talk. I promise to keep the lame jokes to a minimum; you won't have to look at the paintings. There is a pathway near the hospital next door that is pleasant enough and we can talk. We can decide from there what to do."

For a moment she softened, letting go of her tough-girl attitude. It was the first time her shoulders dropped and she looked at me rather than through me: a window of hope.

"So if we are outside, I can smoke, right?"

"Sure."

In the past I had worked with patients with agoraphobia and was willing to go out with them to different places as part of helping them desensitize. But I had never done an outside session as a way to keep myself from throwing up.

I walked back down the hall to the group room, and told Dolores I would be back within the hour. She shook her head and gave me one of her no-nonsense looks. Dolores was protective of me, and when I did something that she thought was unnecessary or risky, she let me know.

The sullen teenager used the walk to lay out the puzzle of her life. Piece by piece she offered clues. She spoke for a half hour as I nodded my head and punctuated her comments with "uh-huh" and "I understand," and when she was finished I repeated her story back to her in my own words, to make sure I hadn't missed anything.

Suzanne's life was a train wreck. Her father had been a physically abusive alcoholic and had broken her jaw during a beating when she was seven. He'd died when she was eight and her brother was four. Her mom became alcoholic after that and started bringing men home from bars.

"She would let anybody fuck her," Suzanne said. "I was only ten years old and I could see these guys were scum bags."

When her mother ran out of money she moved to Newark, began prostituting, and started using heroin. By the time Suzanne was thirteen things were worse than ever.

"We were the only white people in the neighborhood and my mother was fucking men for money. If she had a John inside she would leave a red ribbon tied around the front door knob.

I'd come home from school and there would always be a fucking ribbon. That's what my friends and me called it, actually. The *fucking* ribbon. If it was on the door, my mother was fucking. After a while I just stopped coming home. I'd call her to tell her whose house I was staying over, and she would scream at me for bothering her. Nice, eh?"

"What happened with your brother?"

"He got hurt at school—some kid punched him in the eye and he nearly went blind, and after that my grandmother took him in and he went to school down here, the good ol' Jersey Shore."

"Then things changed."

"Yeah, my mother found God or whatever, and she became a Jehovah's Witness."

"That was when she stopped drinking and cleaned up her act, so to speak."

"Yeah, but then she was dragging me door to door with the fucking *Watchtower* magazine to save people. How fucking stupid is that? They think that one hundred and forty-four thousand people are going to be saved—and these stupid bastards keep recruiting people and boast that they have millions of followers worldwide. It didn't seem like a good bet for me to join some loser group that says no matter what the fuck you do only a hundred forty-four thousand are going to be saved—and I figure if you just joined, there are millions of people ahead of you, so what are the chances you're going to beat them out and become one of the chosen few? Not very good, I'd say."

We had reached the end of the path.

"Why don't we turn here and head back?" I suggested. "So, we were up to the Jehovah's Witnesses."

"Hallelujah!" she said as she turned on her heel.

"Right. Then your mother meets Frank."

"Fucking Frank."

"Frank has a lot of money and starts coming over regularly and your mother is off the drugs and booze and has found God."

"When Frank started coming over I thought we had hit the fucking lottery. He brought my mother flowers; he brought me little things of candy and stupid stuffed animals. I was fourteen and we had been through so much shit that this guy seemed like a prince. He owned like ten video shops or something like that."

"So, Frank lived down here at the good ol' Jersey Shore, and one of his shops was up in Newark. Then he invited you and your mother to live with him down here."

"It was like something out of a movie. He had this great house just off the beach. It was a fairy tale."

"So for a couple of years until you were sixteen, things were good. You made friends, did well in school; in fact you were in the gifted and talented program and scored really high on the standardized tests. Then, in the last semester of your junior year, that's when you found the tapes Frank made with the hidden camera."

Suzanne stopped walking. I could see her bottom lip quivering. Her face suddenly appeared from behind the mask, and her eyes filled up. She wasn't some tough, streetwise homeless teenager, she was a little girl. She covered her face, but her hands seemed too small to do the job, and tears leaked out from under them.

I had forgotten to bring any tissues and tried to offer words for comfort.

"I know this must be painful for you to talk about. Maybe we can just walk back to the office. We don't have to talk about this anymore. You did a lot today."

She shook her head up and down in short bursts, agreeing with me.

"I didn't know all this shit bothered me so much. Christ I need a cigarette," she said.

She took out a Marlboro Light, lit it, and tried to shake off the feelings.

"How do you listen to all this crap? How many people do you see in a day? After listening to all this stuff all day long, what do you do—go home and fuck the cat? How is any of this going to help, anyway? You must get off on listening to other people's screwed-up lives."

"The truth is I just try to really listen and understand it. My cat-fucking days are pretty much over."

She burst out laughing. It was the kind of laugh that was too much of a reaction: she needed the release. So did I.

She finally took a deep drag on her cigarette and held it in for a long time. When she let it out she started walking again. We were almost back at my office.

"I admire you for being able to talk about everything you did today," I offered.

"Christ, I'm tired."

"That makes sense," I responded.

"How come?" she said, looking at me through swollen eyes.

"When you have to hold in so much information and feeling, it takes a lot of energy. When you finally talk about it, it's like a log jam has burst and all the pent-up energy is released."

Her eyes moistened again.

"So what do we do now, good doctor?"

"What do you want to do?"

"I don't know. I mean, I had so much fun today, I don't know how I could go on without . . ."

She started to cry again. This time it was unbridled and she sobbed into her hands. I was glad we were the only ones on the path and she could let herself cry. After a minute she calmed herself, and began to laugh.

"This is like some kind of fucking drug!" she blurted out. "My head is spinning, there is so much going on. I can't believe I am crying like some two-year-old."

She tossed the cigarette on the ground and stepped on it.

"What I can tell you is that you did an incredible amount of work today on letting go of the pain and trying to make sense of all the shit that has happened in your life," I told her. "I really mean it when I say I admire you. I'm impressed with your resilience and your courage."

"Yeah, well, that's the kind of chick I am. I was voted most likely to be resilient."

"You don't have to decide now what you want to do. You can call me during the week and let me know what's what."

"Right, I have to check my schedule and everything," she said sarcastically.

"Of course," I said.

"What would we talk about next time? Maybe this is it, right? Maybe I told you all of the nasty stuff and that's that."

"Well, I think I would start with your nickname. How come they call you Cutter?"

She looked at me for what seemed to be a long time, but it could only have been a few seconds. It was as though she were deciding if she wanted to tell me. She stayed focused on my eyes and unbuttoned her coat and let it drop to the ground. She unbuttoned the left cuff of the long-sleeve green-checked flannel shirt she had on. She never took her eyes off of mine. When the button was undone she pulled the cuff up, just to the bicep, to reveal a galaxy of micro, inch-long slashes all up her arm. She broke her gaze with me and stared at her arm briefly, then covered it and buttoned her cuff. She bent down, picked up her coat and put it back on. As she arranged herself her eyes met mine again.

"I think I can make room in my schedule for one more go around. I'll see you same time next week."

"Same time," was all I could get myself to say.

. . .

For months we met fifteen minutes after Dolores left on Wednesdays, and Suzanne showed faithfully, arriving a few minutes early for each session. Over the course of our conversations, I learned more of her story.

Prince Frank had hidden cameras recording Suzanne in the shower, having sex with her boyfriend, and masturbating. He was selling them as porn to chosen customers in his shops. The day she took the Midol was the day someone left the video in her high school locker.

Afterward, Frank left, and her mother turned back to prostitution, drugs, and abusive boyfriends. She blamed Suzanne for Frank leaving, and for "ruining my life" by making a big deal out of the videos.

In the nineties, the grunge music and the anti-fashion scene had migrated from the Seattle area and caught on with what my colleague called "denigration X" in Jersey. After the Midol incident, Cutter, a name I never called her, dropped out of high school and took up the grunge attitude and look. At the end of one of our walks, I watched as Suzanne got into what she called her "diarrhea-brown" Toyota. The grunge mantra on her bumper sticker said it all: *I don't care what you think of me* was unevenly glued on the trunk.

But the truth was, Suzanne also didn't care much about herself.

After dropping out of school, she began cutting herself daily, and found, surprisingly, that it made her feel better. Over months of therapy I learned that she made cuts when she was depressed, angry, or, on rare occasions, happy. She didn't do drugs, didn't care for alcohol, didn't have a boyfriend or a girlfriend, and painted with oils or watercolors every day.

But despite what I was learning about her, therapy wasn't working. As our sessions continued, her hygiene improved only slightly and, as the weather turned toward the warmer months and her coat was shed in favor of long-sleeve shirts, I began noticing spots of fresh blood through her left sleeve.

When I made a contract with her that stated she would not attempt to kill herself, she signed it. Her only remark was: "Whatever."

By the fall, she admitted she liked coming and "talking about all the crap in my head," but after six months of weekly sessions nothing had improved. She was still cutting herself, gouging homemade tattoos, and making herself look distinctly unattractive. This took some doing as her innocence and simple beauty seemed always present. It was as though the child in her were waiting to be discovered again. It was hard for me to watch her disfigure herself. It seemed as if she were deliberately trying to repulse me and drive the world away.

In October, she greeted me with her left wrist out, face up, with the letter *F* poked into her skin. "I made it this morning," she said with mock pride. "F is for Frank, fucking Frank. F is for failure. F is for fuck you, fuck me, and fuck everybody. F is for fuggedaboutit, F is for . . ."

"I get it," I said, intentionally interrupting her.

"Don't you like my new tattoo?" she said. "I'm thinking of doing the whole alphabet."

I opened the door leading out of the waiting room and we began walking over toward the hospital. The tattoo and her question undid me. Sideswiped, my mind was now whirling. Her centripetal depression was pulling me in.

Her flagrant disregard for herself, her charismatic but abrasive personality, the self-destructive bent but the refusal to miss an appointment, the cursing, the smell, the ink, the blood, her brown eyes, youth, artistry, the lousy parenting—all reminded me of my cousin, his tattoos. "Don't you like my new tattoo?" he'd say—his fucking addiction, the night he died, he overdoses, I am helpless, he is dead.

Gary grew up on MacDougal Street in New York's Greenwich Village with his alcoholic parents. He was my second cousin, but we grew up like brothers. Even as a kid I realized there was something wrong with his parents. They had doughy gray skin and their vein-popping eyes looked like roadmaps to nowhere. They said and did stupid things; his father got loud and his mother fell asleep. They lived in their own fucked-up world and always smelled like scotch—or wine, or beer, or whatever was open—and Romano cheese.

I was jealous of him because he was offered a full scholarship to NYU to study filmmaking. He never seemed to study, drank every day, and didn't have to pay for his education. Me? I had to bust my ass for everything.

But he dropped out of NYU in his first semester, after he found pot, cocaine, and heroin. He shot up with everybody: big-time actors, small-time crooks, guys in the mafia, rock stars, hookers, and the other junkies in Washington Square Park.

As I walked with Suzanne that day, a terrible memory came back to me.

I am at Gary's funeral. Last night we were at a party; the next evening he's in a coffin. Shot too-good heroin into that new tattoo. I should have known. Didn't want to know. He had to do the most drugs, be the worst, die the youngest. A front-row seat to his self-destruction. Couldn't save him. Graduate school. I'll save everybody else.

"I can't do this anymore," I began as we walked. "Therapy isn't working. I can't watch you destroy yourself. I can't watch you poison yourself right in front of me."

I wasn't even looking at her. I just kept walking and talking.

I explained that I was at a loss about how to help her. This shocked her, but I was the one who was most surprised. The countertransference resulting from my memory of my cousin had blindsided me. She was him. He was always getting new tattoos to hide the track marks; he had a miserable childhood and was as bright as could be—and as self-destructive. I had watched him die; I wouldn't watch her. There was a long moment when she knew I was serious about ending the therapy. I could see she was considering telling me something.

"I bet you want to know why I do all this," she said as she gestured down the length of her torso with her hand.

"Yes, I do."

"I do it to control people," she said. "I know that when I walk into a room I'm controlling everyone's reaction. They look at me and they are grossed out. I *make* them feel that way. I *make* them feel sick to their stomachs when they look at me. No one rejects me—I *cause* them to react. I don't wait for their approval—I force them to reject me; that gives me control. My mother hates it too—that means I have control over how she feels about me. I master my own world."

Suzanne was Gary: be the worst, die the youngest.

She had given me an opening. I took a chance.

"I can't believe it," I said. "I never would have thought that about you. Of all the things I would have labeled you as, I would never have labeled you as something as unadventurous as a reactionary-conformist, someone controlled by others' reaction to them. A slave, not a master."

"What! A slave? A reactionary?" She bristled. "I just told you *I control* those people. *I* make them feel that way towards me! How do you see that as being a slave?"

"You don't control them," I said, stopping and staring into her eyes, "*they* control *you*. You *have* to be the ugliest, smelliest, most repulsive person in the place. You don't have free will: you *have* to be the one they reject. You've given all your power to them. You're not free to decide who you want to be—you're so busy trying not to be them that you don't take the time to figure out who you really are, who *you* want to be. All you are interested in is not becoming them."

"All you shrinks are fucked up," she said, grinding her cigarette into the ground. "I've had enough of this bullshit. You're right— you're not helping me one fucking bit. I finally tell you what's going on with me and you make this stupid-ass interpretation. Well you're wrong, *I* control them, and if you can't get that, then *I* am out of here."

Suzanne walked off the path. She lit another cigarette right after she turned her back on me. Her walk was a deliberate trudge. She inhaled and blew out smoke in rhythm with her fury: a runaway train.

She cut across the lawn to her car and I yelled to her.

"Same time next week," I blurted out in desperation.

She stuck the middle finger of her right hand up in the air and kept walking away.

What had I just done? Had Gary's death just fucked up what I did with a patient? What the hell was I doing? This was a borderline patient or, more specifically, a borderline-borderline; she didn't even meet the full diagnosis, but had many of the characteristics. Technically she was splitting on me—I had just gone from the good guy to the asshole. Borderlines don't know about the colors gray or beige. Everything and everyone is either black or white, good or bad. But more worrisome: had I gotten caught in the swamp of her psyche, and was I splitting on her? She had gone from the one I was going to save—to the one I wouldn't work with. I was lost.

The week was hell. I wanted to call her, but instead got hold of my old supervisor. We talk endlessly about what was going on, what I should do, and whether I should call Suzanne. The decision was to wait.

She showed up fifteen minutes early for her next appointment. Usually we met outside the building, but today she came in just as Dolores was getting ready to leave. I was relieved to see her: no, I was overjoyed. She sat on the couch in my waiting room with clean hair, wearing a pair of black jeans and an oversized white long-sleeve tee shirt. No crummy coat, no layers, no smell.

Dolores eyed her up and down, and then glanced back at me. This wasn't lost on Suzanne.

"Don't gloat," she said to both of us. "It's just too cold outside. I thought it was time to move the circus inside."

"Inside," I said, "is a very good place for us to go."

....

Dan Tomasulo holds a PhD in psychology, an MFA in writing, and a master in applied positive psychology from the University of Pennsylvania. In addition to teaching at New Jersey City University, he works with Martin Seligman, "The Father of Positive Psychology," at Penn. He blogs for Psychology Today, Psych Central, *and* Answers.com, *and Sharecare has honored him as one of the top ten online influencers on the topic of depression.*

PARADISE/LOST

Jennifer Lunden

"When you're a therapist, you learn how not to react . . . even when they say things that strike you as absurd," observes a clinical social worker. Yet, to the author's surprise, her gradual willingness to share her own thoughts and opinions makes all the difference to her client, a young woman struggling to trust her own perceptions of the world.

I don't know why it is that when I try to describe Astra, what comes to me first is her hair. It was long, straight, and brown, like mine was before I got it cut into this short, professional cut, before the gray came in. She wore a battered brown felt hat in that first session—probably well loved and well kept by its first owner, and then loved in a looser, more casual way by her. Her shirt and vest looked to have been found at the bottom of the bargain bin at a funky thrift shop, and also like they had been picked up off the floor and assembled on her body in a hurry.

That first day, she hung her head in such a way that her hair often obscured her face. But later, when she trusted me, she revealed more of herself. Sometimes, there was great suffering in her hazel eyes; sometimes, an impish twinkle.

It's impossible to show the complexity of a narrative in a short essay. I cannot tell all parts at once. How do I choose which part of the story to tell? And what order should I impose? How do I do justice to Astra's complex story? Or should I say, her multiple, intertwined stories?

In our second-to-last session, when I introduced the idea of writing this piece about her, Astra was enthusiastic. And before I could explain something I thought was important, she said it first: "I know that the essay will be *your* version of my story, and different from mine."

In our first session she told me that she had dropped out of college two years earlier. She spent a few months living with friends and eating their food, feeling lost, feeling crazy. Then she came here to Maine—"for asylum," she said. She moved into her grandmother's garden shed, and took a job as a cook in a pub.

"I don't know . . ." she said. "I've always been highly sensitive. I get really happy, and then I get really sad, back and forth throughout the day, and I'm anxious, and sometimes I have panic attacks, and I kind of feel like I'm in a fog all the time, and I'm not *doing* anything."

"What would you *like* to be doing?" I asked.

"I'd like to be contributing to the world in some creative way. But I'm having a hard time narrowing it down. I have difficulty focusing. I think I may have ADD."

She expressed ambivalence about her sexuality, and said she was tired of thinking about it, because her thoughts and experiences had been so circular. She had come out at fourteen, and had had a number of lesbian relationships, but was now seeing a man named Hamm. They were not exclusive, and she frequently wound up sleeping with other men and women. "But that's okay," she said. "I don't subscribe to conventions. What's confusing is that I get a sense of peace when I think about being single, but then there seems to be some kind of compulsion to be with people." She thought for a moment. "I feel really messed up, but I don't feel like there's any good reason for it. I grew up privileged."

I asked her about her parents.

"My mom seems normal," she said, "but she's emotionally closed off and robotic. My dad is more accessible, but he's moody. But they're both good people," she was quick to interject. "I don't know what's wrong with me . . . Do you think meds might help, for the ADD, I mean?"

I explained to Astra that I'm a licensed clinical social worker and not qualified to prescribe meds. I told her about a piece I'd read in the *New York Times*, which indicated that stimulant treatment for ADHD helps only in the short run and may cause lasting changes in the brain.[*] The mainstream media could provide any number of narratives in favor of medications for ADHD, but I felt it was important to offer Astra other perspectives. So I also suggested she read the chapter on ADHD in Robert Whitaker's *Anatomy of an Epidemic*. Whitaker refers to one meta-analysis that found little evidence that stimulants improved academic performance. And he cites another study, by the National Institute of Mental Health, in which the researchers conclude that "the long-term efficacy of stimulant medication has not been demonstrated for *any* domain of child functioning."[†]

"I'm not a doctor," I said, "and I'm not saying you shouldn't take those meds. But there might be some other options. For instance, many people have found changes in diet can help."

Astra admitted she often forgot to eat, adding that she had had "numerous freakouts" from not eating, so she tried, now, to eat more regularly—"but the less you eat, the harder it is to remember."

....

[*] L. Alan Sroufe, "Ritalin Gone Wrong," *New York Times*, January 28, 2012, http://www.nytimes.com/2012/01/29/opinion/sunday/childrens-add-drugs-dont-work-long-term.html?pagewanted=all&_r=0.

[†] Robert Whitaker, *Anatomy of an Epidemic: Magic Bullets, Psychiatric Drugs, and the Astonishing Rise of Mental Illness in America* (New York: Broadway Paperbacks, 2010), 225–26.

She denied that she had ever had an eating disorder. But then she said, "If I feel really full or eat something bad, I will make myself throw up." She told me she did this perhaps twice a month. "But I don't want you to think it's any big deal. It's not a big deal."

There was something cagey about Astra. She would touch on a subject—her parents, her sex life, her eating—and hint that there was something wrong, but then she would flip her story and tell me there was nothing wrong at all. I couldn't blame her for resisting being pathologized. Who wants to be pathologized? So when she told me she had a privileged life, I went with it, although I suspected the truth was much more complex; and when she told me she was okay with her indiscriminate sexuality, I went with that, too. Now, when she told me about making herself vomit, I worried about anorexia. But I knew that pursuing it any further would only cause a retreat. Our first work together was to build trust. Which meant that I needed to honor what she had to say. I needed to not dig too much.

In our fourth session, Astra described a lifelong lack of "stick-to-it-iveness" which had lead to creative paralysis. "I get disenchanted with projects I was excited about and then just stop."

This, I knew, was a symptom of ADHD. But when Astra explained that she began to lose interest in projects the minute she started them, it was clear to me there was more to the story, and I asked her about it.

"I'm too hard on myself," she said. "I don't think I have anything of value to offer as an artist. I think it's selfish and indulgent to do art."

When you're a therapist, you learn how not to react, how to sit with someone from your center, even when they say things that strike you as absurd.

"Has anyone else's art ever been of value to you?"

"Well . . . yes," said Astra. "I'm very paradoxical. I view the world paradoxically. It's why I have a hard time doing things sometimes."

Astra told me that every day she sat down and made a list of things to do, and then she got carried away researching new things and ideas, and then everything got too daunting and she got overwhelmed and didn't do anything. It was clear to me that Astra was paralyzed by the symptoms of ADHD. But why? Was it as simple as needing a prescription for Adderall? I gave her the names of a psychiatrist and a naturopath who specialized in alternative treatments for ADHD, but she never called them.

Together, we brainstormed a list of things that helped alleviate her ADHD symptoms. The list included sleeping eight hours every night; eating consistently, making sure to eat healthy foods and get enough protein; taking supplements such as vitamin B12 and fish oil; exercising; using her creativity; being in the woods; and having some routines. Then we came up with a plan of small, manageable goals for the upcoming week.

The next time we met, she told me she had followed the plan "knowing it was something I had to do, not something I wanted to do, but when I started feeling good, I wanted to do it more." She gained weight and felt more clearheaded, and she thought her moods might have been better.

However, she noted that she resisted routine. "Any time there's a system, I feel like it's brainwashing me. I spend a lot of my days avoiding things."

And that's how it went with Astra. She would hit on something that worked for her, and then she would slip. One day, I asked how she was doing with food and exercise, and she expressed frustration with that question. "That's not living to me!" she said. "I get bogged down in the day-to-day maintenance. Cooking and eating three meals a day, exercising, showering . . . they take so much energy. They make me want to give up. It's hard to follow through and finish things."

"Those day-to-day maintenance things are the *foundations* for you to be able to have a clear mind, be able to follow through with things, and feel good about yourself, Astra," I said. "And from what you've told me, you aren't really living *now*," I added, challenging her.

Astra smiled. "You're right. My body gives me messages, but I don't want to hear them. Like, if I don't get enough sleep for even one night, it's guaranteed I will have a panic attack or crying fit."

The next time we saw each other, Astra said she liked it when I had been more assertive. We discussed the pros and cons of this approach. I expressed my frank concern that she had such difficulty knowing her own identity, I didn't want my opinions and perspectives clouding her own. However, she felt confident that she could make her own sense of things. She added, "And if I feel like you're holding back, I might share less."

So I began sharing my thoughts and opinions more freely, and sure enough, our sessions became more alive, more dynamic.

"I'm so fed up with myself. I'm like this dog that's never been trained. I feel like a puddle." Astra sat across from me, rumpled and discouraged.

"You *are* kind of a puddle right now," I said. I decided to share something personal. "There was a time in my life when I was a puddle, too. Some of us who feel torn down by life have the opportunity then to build ourselves up anew, and that is what I see you beginning to do."

Astra put her head down and wept. "I don't even know why you like your job," she said.

It seemed like a strange thing to say in that moment, but I knew what she meant. *Why would you want to spend so much time with messed-up people like me?* "I like it because I see people get better," I said. "And if you stick with it, I have no doubt that you will be amazed at the progress you make. These basic things we are working on right now, like eating regularly, are building the foundation for the amazing things I think you're going to do in your life."

"Really?"

"Really."

As she was leaving, I asked Astra if she needed me to write down her next appointment time on a card. "No," she said. "I'll remember. I look forward to this. I have been looking for you for a long time."

What a sweet thing, this relationship that was building between us.

It seemed that whenever Astra talked about her sex life, there was a new lover. There was Hamm, and later there was Hamm's roommate. There was an actor. There were men and women she met at work.

The ADHD even appeared to manifest in her sexual choices.

"I was raised in a sex-positive environment," she said. Later, she spoke of her bisexuality: "I'm a rogue, a nomad, straddling two worlds." Her eyes twinkled mischievously. "I'm not going to let the straight world tell me what I can do."

Once day, however, she began to weep. "I feel like people just want to sleep with me," she said. "It gets to the point where it feels like that's what I'm good for."

As she lamented her lack of friends, I asked about May, a new friend she had recently mentioned with excitement. Now, however, Astra folded into herself, her hair falling into her face. "I had sex with her boyfriend," she said, "so I've been avoiding her. But it's no big deal."

"You say it's no big deal," I said, "but your whole body closed down just now."

"It's no big deal because it doesn't mean anything," she said. "But I've been betrayed in relationships. I know how it feels. I don't regret most of the people I have sex with, but I regret having sex with May's boyfriend, even though it wasn't a big deal and nothing was meant by it."

One day, I asked Astra to tell me more about what it meant to be raised in a "sex-positive" environment. She said, "Sex was very important. But now I realize there was no room for me to decide for myself what I thought and felt about sex. My mom and her friends were always talking about their 'sexcapades.'"

I flashed to my own childhood. My mother at the ironing board suddenly telling me about sex, although I hadn't asked: "I had to learn about sex by watching the bull mate with the cows in the pasture," she said. "I don't want it to be like that for you. You can ask me anything."

How I stood awkwardly in the doorway, wanting to turn on my heels and go.

My discomfort when she walked around the house naked.

That day in the kitchen when she told the eleven-year-old me about how she had never had an orgasm until she was an adult, and she had never masturbated until she was encouraged by a therapist to do so.

And later, when I was twenty, when she insouciantly mentioned the affairs she'd had while she was married to my father.

"One time," said Astra, "on my twelfth birthday, I convinced my parents to let my boyfriend stay overnight. He slept in my bed, and we did 'everything but.' I begged them to let me, but it actually didn't feel very good. I wish they had said no."

"Kids are always asking for more," I said. "But in reality what they want more than anything is for their parents to hold safe boundaries. It sounds like you feel they didn't do that for you."

"Yeah. We were too young. It was kind of gross. Now, I think of sex like dancing. It's just something that feels good and is fun to do with another person. The problem is that there often tend to be human entanglements that complicate things."

She wondered if the sexuality she sensed in people was actually creativity, and said she wanted to transform her sexuality into creativity, "wild and irreverent."

Astra strongly believed her destiny lay somewhere other than Maine. "I feel like there's a pool of friends waiting for me somewhere. But I'm afraid if I move I won't find a job and I'll be homeless, down and out, depressed, or in jail."

So for the time being, she stayed.

"My mother thinks I'm a spoiled baby, and naturally fucked up," Astra said early in our time together. Her voice wavered with emotion.

"And that's what you fear about yourself, isn't it?" I said.

Astra broke into tears. She nodded. "I've always felt rejected by my mother, but my mother always says that she felt rejected by *me*." Then she said, "A friend in college gave me a book on narcissistic mothers, but I didn't know what to think. It's confusing, because my mother is also very sweet."

"When you're the daughter of a narcissistic mother," I said, "there's a special kind of enmeshment that happens. It's hard to distinguish who you are separate from your mother."

Astra looked up at me. The tears fell down her face. "I have the feeling that there's something *nasty* about me, and I don't know what it is. I don't like my mother that much. I don't like it when she touches me."

That word, *nasty*, had such strong connotations of sexual shame, I couldn't help but wonder if she had been sexually abused. Just as I was about to ask, Astra said, "I don't think I was sexually abused. I don't have any memories of anything like that. But it was a drinking culture at our house, and it always felt like I was on a rocking boat. I grew up in a touchy-feely culture, with people touching me when I didn't want them to, but it wasn't sexual abuse. . . . I really do feel like there is something fundamentally *wrong* with me. I feel *fundamentally bad*."

There was nothing about Astra that seemed bad to me. Her worst problem, as far as I could see, was an overwhelming shame, a lack of trust in her own perceptions, her own validity, her own place in the world. I knew what it was like to lack trust in one's own perceptions. I, too, had had a mother who denied my experience of reality. I, too, had felt rejected by a mother who told me it was I who had rejected her.

I asked Astra for some examples of how she was fundamentally bad, and she said, "Sometimes I don't care about people's feelings. I have a sadistic sense of humor. I am mischievous. I've hurt people."

That was it? I sat forward in my chair and said, "Astra, you are *not* fundamentally nasty. That is a shame word that has to do with your past experiences and not with who you are. Those are examples of very human behavior, some of it committed by a human who is uncertain about how to be in the world and how to do relationships."

Astra sighed a big sigh of relief. Tears welled up in her eyes. She said, "My mother takes on a role of victim in life, so I'll always be the evil one."

Soon after, Astra came in eager to share a powerful dream she had had the night before. In it, she was walking through woods. It was a beautiful spring day and all the colors were electric. She felt cradled by a canopy of leaves, and was walking on soft moss. She came upon a little house that was camouflaged by trees. Inside, the house was creaky, dusty, moldy, decomposing. She walked into the back of the house and found an emaciated woman in the bedroom—pale, with a bloated, malnourished stomach. "She's just a body and the skin is hanging on her," said Astra. The woman's eyelids were heavy, and Astra couldn't tell if she was looking at her or not. "I felt strangely at home. I picked her up and carried her out."

Astra smiled. "I think that woman is me! I think this dream is about my efforts to make myself happy."

I smiled, too. "I agree. I think your dream is about this work we are doing in counseling. I think you are going to that old, decomposing house and rescuing yourself."

One day, we talked about how hard it was for her to speak badly of her family. She rushed to say, "There are a lot of beautiful things about my childhood and my parents. My mother's best friend Andrea used to always say, 'You're so spoiled. Be grateful.'"

I said, "I don't believe there is a fundamental truth; just all of us with our various truths. My hope for our work is that we can find a way to put what is beautiful in a certain place of the room and acknowledge that it is there, but that you can also give yourself permission to explore your own truth, even if it is not others."

Two weeks later, she struggled to overcome her guilt as she spoke of aspects of her childhood that troubled her. She said, "In our family, I was seen as the little Scorpio child. Scorpios are notorious for being sexual, and from a young age, I was sexualized through that framework. When I was going through puberty, Andrea and my father told me to be proud of my tits and show them off. Later, Andrea and I had open discussions about everything; she would tell me about her 'sexcapades.' My parents also talked about theirs. When I would say, 'This is wrong,' they brushed me off. I always felt like a goody two-shoes."

Astra had a look of disgust on her face, and I asked her what feelings were there for her. She said, "Disbelief and irritation. When I look at myself as a little girl, I get pissed off I had to deal with it. I'm really angry. But at the same time, I feel guilty. People always told me, 'You grew up in paradise.'"

When I asked Astra if she would like to talk about the things that were good about her childhood, she started weeping. "My parents are some of the kindest people I know. My mom taught me to read when I was four by putting notes all over the house that would say what things were. So a rug would say 'rug,' and a plant would say 'plant.' My dad is a carpenter. They made me a tree house. My dad believes in karma and gave his van to a newlywed couple. Andrea's door is always open and she cooks for people and they give back. It's a gift culture."

I asked Astra if she knew why she was crying, and she said she didn't.

"It sounds like the loss of a garden of Eden."

"Yes, that's it," she said. "But I don't want to go back there."

In our next session, Astra said, "I've been thinking a lot about things since our last session. I can't tell if I lost something good or I escaped something bad. I make a pretty story, I make an ugly story."

"It's hard for you to trust your own perception," I said.

"I want the more romantic image of my childhood to be true. Self-editing keeps me from going down into my own depths. It keeps things superficial."

A few weeks later, Astra told me she gets "icy" around her mother but then feels guilty.

I thought about it a moment, and then decided that my self-disclosure would be beneficial to Astra. "When I was thirty-six, my mom came to visit, and for some reason I didn't understand at all, I felt myself cringing in her presence. I felt an *aversion*. I froze up around her. It was protective; my body gave me no choice. I felt like a terrible daughter. I tried to hide it, but she could feel it. She asked me about it. I told her I didn't know why it was happening, and that I was sorry. I asked her to give me some space. We didn't have much contact for a long time. In my own therapy, it became clearer, with time, that my mother didn't have a good sense of boundaries. I grew up feeling invaded, but whenever I expressed my discomfort, she dismissed my feelings. Like you, I felt like I was a goody two-shoes."

"Thank you for telling me that story," said Astra. "It helps."

One day, discussing her difficulty committing to an exercise regimen, Astra explained, "I need structure because I am too chaotic. The problem is that when I make these decisions, it feels like an autocratic voice inside me, and then a rebel part comes out to contend with the autocrat." I told Astra that a therapeutic modality called Internal Family Systems holds that we're all made up of parts. I said some of the work in therapy is to help the parts work together more compatibly. Astra liked this concept very much, but when I explained that the belief is that there is a core self as well, she objected, "I don't think anything has an essence. I believe we're all vessels and stuff flows through us."

"How does this belief serve you?" I asked. I knew it was a challenging question. But previously, Astra had told me of her spiritual confusion—her desire to have a spiritual framework, but her deeper underlying sense that the world is essentially absurd and meaningless. Her belief that nothing had an essence struck me as a big part of her sense of rudderlessness.

"That's a good question," said Astra. "I know I am very influenced by my own philosophies but I don't realize it. I feel like I have one foot in the world and one foot out of it, so I don't feel very active and involved. It's just pretend. But not being proactive is killing me."

One day, Astra told me that she had been saving up for a weeklong residential workshop in physical theater at a famous performance center. She lit up as she said, "I really am a physical person. I like to perform feats. I always held back from doing anything like this because it's not intellectual. But now I just realized I can't be ashamed of something that comes naturally to me. I feel most truly myself when I'm being silly and goofy and absurd."

I lit up, too. Finally, Astra was moving toward her creative self. I couldn't imagine how this week of immersion in physical theater could *not* be a transformative one for her.

"I feel like it's the beginning of something, this workshop," she said.

"I do, too."

A few weeks later, Astra returned, beaming. "We did exercises to wake the body to be alive to others," she told me. "It felt like my sexual energy transformed into creative energy. There was no pressure other than what I was being in the moment. I was so happy to see an affirmation of my instincts. It was an awakening."

She told me about a metaphor one of the teachers used in class. He said that on the first trip to the moon, the astronauts didn't know exactly how to get there. "They just did it chunk by chunk," said Astra. She added, "There are answers. You don't have to know exactly where you're going or what you're doing."

I shared Astra's joy. This is what I had been trying to teach her. To just take a step, even if she felt she was stepping into the void.

"At the center," she said, with a bemused expression, "everyone was so *clean*. Nobody used drugs, and only one person drank a little. I found the daily structure enormously helpful. So I'm trying to keep that going. I'm finding joy in making sure I take care of myself."

I wouldn't be surprised if I raised both my fists in the air in a happy gesture of triumph.

She told me that while she was at the center she did not allow herself to be distracted by sexual encounters. In fact, she never even mentioned Amos, a man she met there. Later, however, he came to visit her, and she told me about him then. He was a professional performer, she said, an organized self-starter. They were well matched in their spontaneity, their creativity, and their intellectual curiosity. She felt safe with him, and the sex was "fantastic." She said, "Spending time with Amos is helping me get a stronger sense of who I am. I always thought of myself as a hippie free spirit because of the way I was raised. But Amos is showing me that it's possible to have some structure in your life and still be a creatively productive person."

Six weeks later, she said, "I used to believe, 'I come from people who drink hard, play hard, and sink hard,' but now I see that

that is a kind of romanticization that has kept me in some messy situations." She thought for a moment, and then she said, "Why did I never notice how badly Hamm treated me?"

"Because at the time, the way he treated you resonated with your beliefs about yourself. But you have changed, Astra."

Astra nodded. "People have noticed. My roommate commented on how much I've changed. It's not that things are solved, but my problems seem more distant now."

We met for our final session a few days before Astra was to fly out of Maine to a new life on the West Coast. The day was bittersweet. "I'm happy for you that you're finally leaving," I said. "But I'll miss you."

We talked about the progress she had made. Astra said, "I play a lot of games—with myself, mostly. But you made me narrow things down and realize I'm creating whatever I create. I realized I had to stop playing games because this is real. I had to get down to a good solid story so I could move forward."

She talked about the pivotal session when she asked me to be more direct about my thoughts, feelings, and biases. She said, "It helped create the foundation where things weren't ambiguous. It was important to know I had a space where you would call me out. I needed a challenge. I needed to know I was talking with someone very human and with real opinions."

As we explored that critical session, I reflected on the ways her childhood felt boundaryless. "It seems like my biases gave you a boundary to push against."

"Yes, that's right. That's exactly what they did."

When Astra was growing up, the adults around her invalidated her experience of the world. This left her confused and ashamed.

To get the love she needed, she developed a system of subterfuge. Her connection to her own knowing went underground— accessible not even to her.

Astra was terrified to say anything against her parents, and that kept her in a paralytic place of shame. My primary job, it seemed to me, was to provide a space where she could acknowledge and process her disowned feelings so that she could heal and move on. That I knew Astra's experience on a visceral level and could share that with her deepened our connection and validated her experience of reality.

As for the ADHD, I don't doubt that Astra suffered the symptoms that could have garnered her a diagnosis. But I also think it's hard to be focused when you are living in a state of shame, unable to acknowledge your own experience, always shrinking in response to the needs of the people around you. When Astra was able to recognize her own truths, that gave her some solid ground to stand on. From there, she could become the author of her own story. She could venture into the world in new ways and give herself permission to care for her brain and her body as they needed.

This is not to say that Astra lived happily ever after. But by the time our work ended, she was finding her way out of her paralysis. She had the tools to build a life of her own choosing.

"I know you still have doubts," I said, as we ended our final session, "but it's obvious to me that you are an artist, and I believe that one day you will come into yourself as an artist, whatever art you decide to do. And I hope you do. Because you have a spark, and I believe that to not do your art would be to deprive the world of that spark."

"I believe that too," said Astra.

I lit up with hope. Was she finally acknowledging the artist inside her?

She explained, backpedaling. "I mean, I believe that all of us have that creative spark."

I laughed. "And I thought you were talking about you, saying that you believe you're an artist."

"I knew you thought that when I saw your face," she said. "That's why I explained." And there it was again . . . that twinkle.

....

Jennifer Lunden, LCSW, LADC, CCS, is a practicing therapist and clinical supervisor, and the founder and executive director of the Center for Creative Healing in Portland, Maine. Her essay, "The Butterfly Effect," won first place in Creative Nonfiction's *Winter 2011 "Animals" issue and went on to win a Pushcart Prize. Named Maine's 2012 Social Worker of the Year, she is also the author of "Salvage, Salvation, Salve: Writing That Heals," which appeared in* Creative Nonfiction *in spring 2013.*

WHAT WOULD MY MOTHER SAY?

Annita Sawyer

Mental health workers often hide their own psychological struggles for fear of damaging their professional reputations. Thirty-five years after her hospitalization as a teenager, one clinician tracks down her medical records and decides to share her story in a bold and memorable way.

"Our deepest fear is not that we are inadequate. Our deepest fear is that we are powerful beyond measure."

—Mariannc Williamson

Shifting from one foot to the other, my back to the stage, I stare at the chattering crowd pouring through the medical school auditorium doors, spilling into empty spaces on the main floor and in the balcony. A red folder and conference brochure claim my front-row seat, but I'm too geared up to take it yet. I note the swelling audience, the din of greetings, shouts, hands waving hello and gesturing, "Come, I saved this one for you."

Here and there, an ill-fitting shirt or a certain stilted gait identifies a psychiatry patient. I know there are others not so easily discerned among the collections of scholars' slacks, psychiatry's black turtlenecks, postdoc jeans, and social worker patterned sweaters. In addition to the usual university students, researchers, faculty, and assorted psychotherapists, this annual Yale conference, presented by the university and the National

Education Alliance for Borderline Personality Disorder, encourages interested patients and their families to attend. Most of the information presented won't be limited by diagnosis, since many serious mental illness symptoms overlap, and diagnostic categories can be arbitrary. I'll be addressing that.

Eventually settling into my seat, I observe a bearded, professorial gentleman plop into the remaining spot on my left. I recognize him from a poster: he's the headliner, the big name draw, who will speak this afternoon. From a weighty briefcase he retrieves a computer he rests on his lap. He begins loading graphs. *I should have worked harder to find photos*, I think.

Eerie calm separates my head from warring jellyfish below my neck. As if my brain is encased in Styrofoam, I remain aware but disconnected from my body's incessant fluttering. Although I've addressed smaller groups in the past, this is the first time I'll tell my story at a national conference. People have paid to attend. I fluff my hair, fiddle with my scarf, count again the pages of my talk.

I've always considered myself a timid person, the opposite of brave. Some of that comes from being shy—feeling stupid and self-conscious among strangers, fumbling for words when I should know what to say. Some comes from absorbing in spite of myself my passive mother's cringing demeanor. *Never put yourself forward*, she taught me. *People won't like you.*

This tendency to shrink from view has also been amplified by shame. As a child in Sunday school I knew I was a worse sinner than my classmates, although I couldn't have told you why. And there was the incontrovertible stigma of being a mental patient for many years, the years when teenagers are making choices about who they are and who they want to be. A half century later, that stigma and its shame still haunt me.

. . .

In 1960, I was suicidal. I saw my death as a way to redeem the shadow my sinfulness cast upon the world. After my parents discovered that I planned to drown myself during a weekend at the beach with high school friends, they admitted me to a psychiatric hospital in my hometown. I had just turned seventeen.

I resisted the doctors' label of schizophrenia, a common diagnosis at the time—I was sure I wasn't interesting enough to qualify—and I hated everything about the electroshock therapy they prescribed: the headaches, the nausea, awaking to the void of not knowing who I was. I approached every ECT convulsion convinced that any miscalculation—an error on the dial, an unanticipated sneeze—would electrocute me. I expected to die. While I schemed to eliminate myself, the prospect of being killed by a random accident terrified me.

Shock treatment made me worse and erased my memory. I developed hallucinations and nightmares and began to bash my head against walls. After three years and countless ECTs I was transferred, "unimproved." When I arrived at the next hospital, I didn't know how many weeks were in a year.

My new doctor and I couldn't connect; we didn't respect one another. Despite wanting a fresh start, I was soon acting out again in increasingly self-destructive ways. I swallowed glass, burned my arms and legs with cigarettes, scratched my face, bit my hands and held them against radiators to burn them. I held my breath until I passed out. I smashed my head against walls, at times requiring stitches in my scalp. I had lost almost all memory of my early years—what remained was only a global sense of fear.

The following year I was assigned to a psychiatrist whose steady centeredness, flexibility, and sense of humor got through to me. When I made stupid puns, he laughed. "What a pain in the neck!" he said once, after I'd smashed my head against the wall. "Spare me," became a running joke between us. If I dared to hint at fears, wrapping them in metaphor, my doctor would respond in kind. He didn't hesitate to send the coast guard to rescue a tiny boat fighting deadly storms at sea. If he appeared upset after I hurt myself, I could tell that his anger came from not wanting me to suffer from more pain.

Over time I grew to understand that everything I did had a reason, and that together my doctor and I could figure out what that was. I no longer felt alone in the universe. I began to see myself as a person instead of an unfortunate syndrome, and this changed my expectations.

As death's urgency diminished, I found new energy for life. "What matters is how well you are, not how sick you are," my doctor was fond of quoting. Knowing that someone I respected believed in me enabled me to achieve beyond what I would ever have imagined alone.

Two years later I left the mental hospital. I found a husband, a bright, troubled seeker like I was, and managed to complete my education. Individual therapies nurtured each of us and, thus, our marriage. Together we raised two children. Sometimes I resented not knowing my own childhood firsthand, but I was very busy and grateful just to be alive.

Gradually, the missing years faded in importance. With a great deal of persistence and good luck I became a clinician myself, determined to pass on the healing psychotherapy that saved my life. But while I did that I kept my past a secret from most of those around me. I certainly didn't tell other psychologists.

You might think that if I was going to risk the stigma that goes with exposing my history in public, a psychiatry conference would be the safest place to do it. Ironically, psychotherapists generally hide these things. Even today, well into the twenty-first century, this blind prejudice might be greatest among mental health professionals. While we dedicate our lives to relieving emotional suffering, accepting and caring for complicated, often difficult, individuals without being judgmental, we fear losing respect and compromising our reputations if we acknowledge this suffering in ourselves.

From my front-row seat I watch the conference director introduce the first speaker, an appealing psychiatrist with wavy dark hair and a gentle voice who tells us how she treats people with complex diagnoses like borderline personality disorder. She describes her patients' sometimes-regressed, flagrantly needy behavior and explains that early unmet needs often underlie these outsized demands for attention. I reflect on my own neediness when I was in the hospital, my driving hunger to feel understood. *Some people love to hog the spotlight, and don't know enough to keep private things private*, I can hear my mother saying. Am I sitting here preparing to tell my story to four hundred people because I love attention and am willing to do anything to get it? I feel my face flush. Sweat spreads across my skin.

Applause breaks my self-absorbed spell. I pat my palms together and nod my head, as if I've been listening all along. The smiling psychiatrist picks up her stack of papers and returns to her seat.

A dozen years ago, I still had no memory of my youth. I had managed a successful psychology practice for decades; my children were grown, my parents long dead. Thirty-five years had passed since my hospital discharge. I decided to send for records from both hospitals to see what I could learn. "Wow. You're brave," said the few friends I told of my plan. "Do you really want to do that?" I felt insulted by their concern.

My doctoral dissertation had focused on clinician bias in psychiatric diagnosis. I showed that things like where the diagnosticians trained and what drugs and treatments were available at the time influenced the diagnoses they chose. Ever since graduate school, I'd used my research to justify dismissing my label of schizophrenia as invalid. I tossed out my extreme behavior as well. *It was the diagnosis du jour, a mistake of the times,* I theorized. *A better diagnosis and a good family therapist would have made all that acting out and hospitalization unnecessary.* Taking pride in my insight, I closed the door on my hospital years. I needed to move forward. I especially needed to avoid getting stuck in resentment for the normal life I had missed.

Brave means ready to face danger; showing courage. Choosing a risky action with uncertain outcome in order to expand one's self-knowledge might qualify. But can a person who is naive and disconnected from the reality of what lies ahead be considered brave? Is she courageous if she ignores the forecast and begins her journey blithely assuming she'll manage, whatever the weather?

My friends were right to sense danger lurking in those records. As a seasoned clinician in 2001 I could easily see what my doctors couldn't in 1960: I'd been suffering from PTSD, not schizophrenia. I recognized evidence of incest that I'd sidestepped for decades: my self-attacks, the biting, burning, cutting, and banging my head against walls; the dissociation, experiencing myself and the world as alien and unreal; my determination to die, not to escape my own pain but to atone for my sins; my father's inebriated fawning. The total of eighty-nine shock treatments—yes, eighty-nine shock treatments!—blindsided me. I was completely unprepared for the reality of my condition.

All the sensations from my disconnected past, which my body had stored since childhood, poured out as terrifying flashbacks: nightmares of dead babies and naked girls, images of body parts just forward of my head, fluttery stomach contractions provoked by certain words or images or thoughts—sex, penis, sin, touch. At night, terror turned my cells to icicles, freezing my core. During the day, writhing larvae infested my limbs.

Retraumatized, I sank into despair in a process I had helped my own patients manage, but couldn't control in my self. I was the meteorologist measuring velocity inside a cyclone that was carrying her away. I resolved that if I survived, I would write about my experience. Again, with skilled help, I recovered.

Indeed, as I grew stronger I began to write. I enjoyed being among writers, in time traveling to workshops far away from home. I discovered that for writers, secrets were just material; pathology intrigued them. Editors' rejections of my early literary efforts kept me humble—and safe. But for a long while, except among writers, I didn't talk about what I was writing.

On stage, the second speaker concludes. A trim, personable neuropsychologist from Canada, he's been describing certain cognitive difficulties identified in people suffering from borderline personality disorder and ways he's devised to measure them. I delight in his accent, especially the sound of his Canadian *o*'s. Although the words themselves hardly penetrate my Styrofoam shell, I enjoy watching him sweep back and forth from the projection screen with his numbers to the audience with his explanations. I join enthusiastic clapping as he exits the stage.

In the brochure, my presentation follows his. All of a sudden I realize that I'm third and it's my turn. This reminds me of my turn for shock—lying flat on a gurney, wrapped in a wet sheet, eyes on the ceiling, advancing slowly down the hall outside the treatment room. *Cool it*, I tell myself.

After a quick introduction, I ascend the stairs, making sure I don't trip, checking at the podium that the microphone picks up the sound of my voice. I smile at the audience. I locate my current therapist, identify several colleagues. *Wow. I can't believe I'm here. Focus!*

A few years ago I was invited to write an article for a special issue of a clinical psychology journal which looked at several senior psychologists' experiences in their own psychotherapy. I was flattered to be asked, so of course I accepted. I enjoyed describing the three intelligent, self-confident, but very different therapists whose work had enabled me to recover. I discussed the many years each therapy had required, and the magnitude of what we accomplished.

Soon after the issue was published, I received my first e-mail from a stranger. "I have only read an online abstract of your piece," she wrote, "but your bravery, and contribution to knowledge, is evident." My immediate reaction, *How cool am I?* was quickly overwhelmed by horror. *I'm ruined! Who'll refer to me now?* Despite the August heat and a patient due, I shut my computer and dashed out the door, racing around the block until I'd calmed down. I had assumed I was writing for a small group of professionals with exclusive access, but it turned out that by Googling me anyone could see the abstract—all of my secrets in a hundred and fifty words. Winded, wiser, I walked home to my office and my patient. *Show-offs always get their comeuppance*, my mother's voice reminded me.

At the conference podium, I'm not halfway through the forty-minute paper before my throat thickens. I've described my experience as a hospitalized teen. I've listed my symptoms, and the way I grew worse until the first hospital gave up. My voice begins to go, scratchy at first. Despite water it gets worse. I sound hoarse. I bite my tongue, a trick I learned in chorus, and it keeps saliva flowing. I push through. *Look at the audience, don't speak too fast, breathe from your diaphragm, you can do this.* To balance the story of damage caused by an inaccurate diagnosis, I describe the doctors who helped me recover, what it means to heal. *Breathe*, I remind myself *You're almost there.*

I lay the stack of pages in front of me and prepare to deliver my last line, skimming it first to make sure I say it correctly. I speak slowly, enunciating every word. This is the message I want to scar into each mind so well that no one present will forget: "It's by setting labels aside, by paying attention to the person right there, and holding yourself open to possibility, that you can save the lives of people like me."

Nothing happens. Silence. I register serious, red faces, wet cheeks, frowns, only a scattering of smiles. No one moves. *I knew it*, I think. *I went too far.* At last someone claps, and it spreads. A man toward the front stands; others follow. The ovation crests like a wave until the entire audience is on its feet.

I observe. I listen. I open my mouth to breathe in the sound, as if I could swallow the air's vibrations, absorb its thunder through my lungs. I want this applause to go on forever, but even more I long for it to touch my heart and autograph my bones, to leave an indelible mark, so I'll know it's real and not a dream. I spread my arms to embrace the now beaming faces, then lower them, then bow my head in thanks.

I return to my seat as the next speaker is introduced. I try to listen, but I really have to pee. The second she concludes I bolt for a ladies' room I noticed earlier just outside the auditorium. By the time I leave its single stall the tiny room is packed with women waiting in line. Sheepishly I return their smiles, nodding thanks to their kind words, still too stunned to speak. By rote I run my hands under the faucet. My wet hand shakes their outstretched dry ones.

Back in the auditorium I'm surrounded by eager, sympathetic faces greeting me with congratulations, thanks, references to my being brave, very, very brave. I keep smiling as I shake more hands.

Among the beaming colleagues, faculty, students, and clinicians of all kinds are those like me who once were, or still are, psychiatric patients grappling with private shame. When we meet our handshakes linger, their eyes lock with mine: *we know*. This is my affirmation. *Nothing else really matters*, I tell myself. I bask in their appreciation, even as doubt rattles inside.

....

Annita Sawyer is a clinical psychologist, in practice over thirty years. Her essays have won awards and been included among notables in The Best American Essays. *Her memoir,* Smoking Cigarettes, Eating Glass, *was selected by Lee Gutkind for the Santa Fe Writers Project literary awards nonfiction grand prize. It will be released in May 2015.*

THE DICTATOR IN MY HEAD

Kurt Warner

Obsessive-compulsive disorder affects about one in one hundred adults. Armed with research and his family's support, one social worker details his ongoing battle against the disorder's relentless commands.

I have a dictator living in my head. Its commands are my earliest memories. It does not care what day it is, what I am doing, or where I am. This tyrant gives me orders endlessly. I awake and it is there, instantly, barking orders at me. Its commands number between five hundred and a thousand per day—a conservative estimate. I once took count—because it makes me count everything, so I thought it'd be clever if I counted it. I lost count around seven hundred commands—and it was around dinnertime. It gives these decrees until I sleep. In fact, the only true escape from the dictator is in sleep. If I don't do what it wants, it makes me feel either intensely guilty, or exceptionally afraid. Fear is its greatest weapon. And the dictator never leaves. Sometimes it gets more powerful and sometimes it gets weaker. But it's always there. This dictator functions on all the same cylinders as the cruel and horrific human dictators throughout history. It uses fear, coercion, and constant threats. It is easiest most of the time just to do what it wants. The problem is that doing what this dictator wants makes it stronger: obeying it is like arming it with more weapons. This dictator, unlike a human dictator, is internal. I cannot escape it, but I have learned how to fight it. I learned this dictator had a name when I was about twelve. Its name is obsessive-compulsive disorder (OCD). Once I learned that, I learned how to fight. Over a lifetime of fighting, I've learned how to live with this internal dictator, and I've come to understand that the power to beat OCD lies within.

According to the National Institute of Mental Health, obsessive-compulsive disorder affects about 2.2 million American adults (1 percent of the adult population). The disorder can be torturous for the millions of people it plagues.

I've been doing battle with OCD at least since I was five years old. I didn't know that the compulsions I felt were a sign of obsessive-compulsive disorder at that young age. OCD manifested itself as counting then, and I had to count every footstep or something horrible would happen. I just did it because I *felt* it was what I had to do. I felt, very strongly, that if I didn't count every footstep, something terrible would happen to my family or to me. So I did it. I counted every footstep by even numbers. One-*two*-three-*four*-five-*six*-seven-*eight*. Then I restarted at one and did it over and over and over. I could not speak while walking or end on an odd footstep. I counted, and counted meticulously. I counted so much that I stopped being conscious of it: my mind automatically counted—the counting actually became so ingrained that I did it without thinking. It became a ritual as ordinary as brushing my teeth. That is an important concept if one is to understand OCD: ritual. Many of the most common manifestations of OCD are inane and absurd rituals. They came to rule my life by the time I was ten.

Slowly, counting my footsteps stopped. I don't recall how or why . . . it just seemed to phase out as subtly as it had phased in. As quickly as counting phased out, the dictator brought a new obsession and accompanying compulsion into my mind. That is the second rule of my OCD: it functions by constant obsession. It is seldom "dormant"— that is, it is like a child who constantly has to have something to do. It finds things on which to obsess, and more than one thing at a time. It is ever busy.

My OCD's second phase (although I still didn't know it was OCD at the time) came to express itself through "checking" various things. I would have to check whether I had locked this, check if I had closed that, and check if I had put everything right where it "needed" to be—because the dictator had a perfect place for me to put absolutely everything on earth. It did not matter that I knew I'd made sure of all these things just a minute ago, either. Over and over and over I had to check them. I checked until there were tears in my eyes. I checked and checked until it "felt" right. Then I could stop. Knowing that the door was locked, the window was closed, and everything in my room was pointing toward the northwest did not matter. Reason was powerless at this point; feeling trumped reason in my mind. My *feeling* that a consequence would occur (for example, that my family would get hurt) would overcome my rationalization that what I was doing was absurd. I could not yet realize that there was no connection between, for instance, checking my desk forty-four times each night to make sure everything faced northwest and was "exactly" right, and my dog not dying. I *had* to check. Usually the checking had to be done, like the footsteps, in even numbers. I learned that the dictator had motifs to its obsessions. Even now it demands even numbers incessantly in my daily life.

The checking phase coexisted with a hoarding obsession. I couldn't give anything away . . . right down to my old clothes, rubber bands, paperclips, you name it. I couldn't get rid of anything because I *felt* that if I did, I would be getting rid of some important part of me. For example, I *felt* that if I gave away my football, my ability to catch would be given away along with it.

The hoarding did not last too long, perhaps a year or so. The checking, however, persists to this day, taking many forms. OCD manifested itself in new obsessions and compulsions constantly. The classic "germaphobia" that popular culture often associates with OCD (such as in the cases of Howard Hughes and Howie Mandel) made a brief appearance. I can vividly remember rubbing my hands on my pant legs so fast and hard they'd burn and get red, tingling in pain. This is how I made them "clean" if I could not get to soap and water. I felt I "contaminated" myself if I put my hands to my mouth after touching something "infected" ("infected" things were very specific . . . like saliva; any saliva was "infected"). If I did get "contaminated," I would "have" to stop swallowing my saliva, and thereby prevent the imaginary germs from entering my body until I could find somewhere to spit, like in a sink or garbage can. One can only imagine how difficult this was (and disgusting). I can remember, in grade school, running to the bathroom as soon as we got a break in class. I would spit saliva that I had been storing up for sometimes thirty minutes or an hour because it was "infected" or "contaminated." It's maddening not allowing yourself to swallow. But OCD made me *feel* that if I swallowed the "infected" spit, I'd get some horrible illness. So the hardship of not swallowing any spit was worth it in my mind.

I can also remember what I call the "good thoughts and feelings" phase of OCD. During this phase, I had to get a good feeling or think a good thought whenever I touched something or did something. If I didn't think a good thought or get a good feeling, I had to repeat the action over and over again until I did. This phase manifested itself in a great many ways. For example, any item I wanted to purchase had to "feel" right to the touch or I could not buy it. I would spend hours in a store feeling one item and then feeling another to see which gave the right feeling.

The counting phase, the checking phase, the germ phase, and the "good thoughts and feelings" phase were not all. There were endless other phases, such as repeating certain phrases in even numbers. These many manifestations of OCD all combined to make every sphere of my life arduous. One example is athletics.

Sports, I found, provided a canvas upon which my obsessions and rituals could paint a hideous picture. People without OCD often perform a multitude of rituals in sports; just think about friends who wear their hats inside out as "rally caps" or refuse to change an article of clothing so long as their team is winning. I found my version of this was like theirs on steroids. I played a lot of sports, in and out of organized leagues, throughout these years. The countless things I "had" to do before each pitch, after every kick, between every play, after—and during—every reception, and in the midst of each serve were utterly exhausting. But, in my mind, it was either do the rituals (compulsions) or lose the game for the team—or worse, much worse. I actually had to quit some teams because it was too overwhelming.

OCD was in the driver's seat of my young life. There was no time that one phase or another of OCD's obsessions and compulsions was not present. There were—and are today— between seven and ten obsessions at any given time. It was only later, in high school, that I began to get it. I noticed that my aunt on my mother's side wouldn't let anyone touch her and wore plastic or latex gloves most places she went. Furthermore, she had not allowed anyone to come into her apartment or her car for the past twenty years, so that no one would contaminate her. My mother's father had to have everything exact and would go into a tirade if his homemade pasta wasn't cut precisely to size. My uncle was a wealthy man but his hoarding was so strong that he would not buy anyone—even family—so much as a cheeseburger at one of the restaurants he owned.

Watching my beautiful but tortured family members struggle motivated me to fight my own false dictator ceaselessly. When I heard talk about something called OCD, I realized I shared many of the experiences of people who had it. I began researching it fervently. I found out that others, countless others, "had" to obey hundreds (and at times thousands) of "orders" given each day by this inner pseudo "master."

Once I became aware—that is, once I studied OCD and realized that what others were battling was very similar to what I was battling—I armed myself with knowledge to fight what I began to see as my inner dictator. I studied the disorder ceaselessly, using credible sources on the Internet and in books. I spoke to others suffering with it through discussion boards devoted to OCD. I knew medications existed (primarily in the form of SSRIs), but I didn't seek medication right away. This was not because I didn't think I could benefit from medication, but because seeking medication would have required telling my parents, and others, such things as that I *felt* certain that if I didn't eat an even number of peas on my plate, my whole family would suffer. Think about telling your family, teachers, and friends that you believe if you don't open and close something seventy-two times, you will lose your girlfriend. I knew it was illogical, and telling people about it seemed, to me, like taking an express route to a sanitarium. So instead, I fought this inner dictator of OCD with knowledge and behavior. I began to understand that the only power it had was its false threats—the imagined consequences of not obeying a compulsion. I started to test it. If I disobeyed its command and drank from someone else's glass, I learned, I didn't get a horrible disease and die a painful death. This knowledge—this *evidence*—enabled me to disobey it constantly because I now knew that it was just lying to me. Through knowledge and trial and error, I learned that it had no real power except to make me feel fearful.

Its power was based on fear . . . and, to paraphrase Franklin Roosevelt: all I truly had to fear was, indeed, fear itself.

Some of the books I read changed my perception of the illness. For example, in *Obsessive Compulsive Disorder: The Latest Assessment and Treatment Strategies*, Gail Steketee and Teresa Pigott explain that the amygdala in the limbic system of the brain is implicated in OCD. This book helped me to see that it was simply an overactive part of my brain or a neurotransmitter imbalance that was causing this nightmare. Learning strategies such as those presented in *Brain Lock* by Jeffrey M. Schwartz and *Stop Obsessing!* by Edna B. Foa and Reid Wilson armed me even more to beat OCD back on a daily basis.

OCD had grown to be a giant in me by this time. There were few if any daily activities during which I was not being "ordered" by OCD to touch this or check that, choose that or do this. I knew full well that I was fighting a dubious battle: I was like David going up against a veritable Goliath called OCD. My sling was the knowledge I had from the books I read, the Internet sites I visited, and the support groups I went to online. And even though it seemed my foe was much more powerful than I, I fought. And as I beat OCD back—that is, as I methodically and routinely disobeyed its orders (compulsions) and ignored its obsessions—I found that it grew clearly and definitively *weaker*. The guilt and shame and fear I felt from disobedience lessened to such a great extent that they did not ruin my day. They still irritated me, changed some of my actions, and absolutely plagued my thoughts. But they no longer controlled me. That, I discovered, was the simple but immutable truth of obsessive-compulsive disorder: to obey its compulsions is to feed it and allow the beast to grow. To disobey its compulsions—that is, to rebel against its orders—is to starve OCD and force it to wither.

Once I discovered this important principle, I began charting the inner dictator's actions. I actually got experimental and cocky and played games with it. I *chose* to feed it when I did not want to suffer the guilt and fear it caused, and *chose* not to feed it when I saw it was getting too strong again. Before long, I thankfully found I no longer *had* to check this, touch that, clean this, and count that. I found what the Doors' lead singer Jim Morrison had said about freedom in general applied in particular to my fight to be free of OCD. He stated, "Expose yourself to your deepest fear. After that, fear has no power, and fear of freedom shrinks and vanishes. You are free." Once I took the leap of rational faith, and disobeyed OCD's irrational rules, nothing bad happened. My dog didn't die, my girlfriend didn't dump me, and my parents didn't get hit by cars. All of its threats were false. My knowledge truly did become my power. I was able to beat the dictator back with a change in behavior. I felt triumphant. I thought I'd won.

However, OCD is Machiavellian. By this, I mean it will do anything to survive. The ends—its survival—justify the means, and there is no end to the variety of shapes it can take in its victim's head. It's sort of like a virus. OCD is truly insidious. As much as I beat it back, it simply found new shapes to take in order to survive. I can remember catching myself almost unconsciously counting the number of words in sentences I wrote, spoke, or heard spoken in order to make sure they ended on an even number, and holding my breath for a certain number of seconds so as not to breathe in during a time when some "bad" thing was occurring (because if I did, OCD made me feel I would "ingest" the badness). What I have found in my many years of battle with this inner tyrant is that OCD can be likened to a leak in a worn hose. That is: if one denies an outlet of OCD's expression, stopping one compulsion/obsession, OCD will find another way to express itself. My point is that the entire realm of the human experience is OCD's canvas . . . it leaves nothing, absolutely nothing, alone. OCD will stop short of nothing to keep itself alive and well. I am naming but a very few of the countless attempts it has made for survival in me.

Despite OCD's strength, through self-education I made incredibly great strides. I was finally able to confide in my mother about it, and she was intensely supportive. I began to tell her what OCD was making me feel, and she helped me to defy it. My mom reinforced my perception that the disorder was genetic and that my other wonderful family members suffered from it, too. I did not feel like I was alone or some kind of freak.

Even though I now benefitted from the support of my family, my OCD continued to find new ways to manifest itself. At the very end of high school and my first undergraduate years, the way OCD found to survive was through what the *DSM IV* calls body dysmorphic disorder (BDD). I found myself utterly obsessed with my appearance. I became convinced that I was completely hideous, despite rational evidence to the contrary. It didn't matter what anyone told me about the way I looked, including girlfriends. I was shocked every day that teachers, friends, and girlfriends didn't scoff at me or run away because I was sure I engendered the same sort of emotional reaction as Joseph Merrick, the "Elephant Man." I would not allow a picture of me to be placed in my high school yearbook, and I would destroy any image of me that I got my hands on. Logic didn't matter. I *felt* it. I felt that my nose was enormous and took up most of my face. I felt that it was my nose that people talked to, not me. And I had to check my appearance constantly. My compulsion was to check myself in every mirror I could find . . . hundreds of times per day. I didn't know how anyone could even look at me for long without being horrified.

However, friends, girlfriends, and relatives *didn't* recoil when they saw me. I was accepted and not rejected by others, and no one made any comments about my appearance. For some time, I thought they were all in collusion, acting like I wasn't hideous out of some Christian impulse of kindness. But, eventually, I caught on. There was a great disparity between the way I *felt* I looked and how others were reacting. Therefore, I went back to books, Internet search engines, and discussion boards. I learned, after a great deal of investigation, about BDD. Although BDD is not necessarily or formally a variant or manifestation of OCD, I can attest to the fact that it was for me.

I could not beat back BDD, despite this knowledge and the reasoning that worked to beat back the other manifestations of OCD. The feelings were too great—or I was just too tired to fight. Therefore, I disclosed the problem and sought treatment. I received psychotherapy and an SSRI. To date, I have tried many psychotropic drugs that can be used to treat OCD but have never found relief from them. I did find the psychotherapy useful because I had another person to help me reason through the obsessions and compulsions. Through therapy, I came to realize that the greatest aid to stopping BDD was learning not to value my appearance so greatly. I realized that appearance isn't everything. Whether I felt I had a nose that took up most of my face or not, I had to live this life. Therefore, I learned not to put all my value on appearance. And it worked. Over time, it starved the obsession. Thus, I beat back BDD as I beat back all the other manifestations of OCD: with knowledge, behavior, family, lots of books, and a good counselor.

Every single one of the aforementioned manifestations of OCD runs on the same basic engine. Each one has an obsession and a compulsion. For instance, my obsession was germs and my compulsion was not swallowing my saliva when I touched something "dirty." My obsession was order and my compulsion was making everything face northwest and locking the doors. Every one of them operates on this basis. After years and years of consciously disobeying OCD's compulsions, I watched it survive by becoming primarily obsessional. Now, it just picks things to obsess on and plagues my mind with them. These obsessions steal sleep from me, and destroy a great many things in my life. At times, I cannot think about much else except these obsessions. It can be very disruptive. For example, I have a good driving record. I constantly drive back and forth between Pennsylvania, where my family lives, and New York State, where I went to graduate school and where I currently work. Near Scranton, Pennsylvania, the two lanes on Interstate 81 narrow for several miles and there are large cement barriers on either side due to roadwork. I began, slowly, over months, to obsess increasingly on the narrowness. OCD persistently flashed images in my mind of crashing my car. Somatic changes occurred: I began to sweat when I'd get near the area and would become overwhelmingly nervous. This occurred for several months before I became *convinced* that I would crash. I had no other option but to take a different route. That new route adds over an hour both ways. That means it cuts two full hours out of the time I can spend every month with my mom. OCD did this through pure obsession.

Another example: about five years ago, I took a medication that resulted in my feeling sick whenever I drink caffeine. The nausea went on for ten months after I stopped the medication and I became very afraid of caffeine. OCD capitalized on this fear. For the last five years, I have been obsessively *terrified* of caffeine. I view caffeine similar to the way Howard Hughes viewed germs. Caffeine contaminates everything for me. My baseball hat recently touched a coffee cup . . . not coffee, but the cup. Ever since, I have been fighting the compulsion to clean it over and over. I get anxiety if someone drinks coffee, eats chocolate, or has some type of tea near me in an enclosed area such as a car.

I find that most of my obsessions wrap themselves like a python around whatever I care about and that my OCD uses those things for the basis of its threats if I do not obey its commands. That is what is so insidious about OCD. It is Orwellian. It chooses what you love most and attacks. Nevertheless, despite this endless mental tyranny on a daily basis, I have been able to live a reasonably normal life. I am happily married. I coordinate a program as a social worker helping individuals suffering from chemical dependency to get back on their feet. I have found that it has helped me to tell good and kind people about my issue with OCD. It makes me feel that I don't always have to conceal it. I have found that concealment and isolation are the breeding grounds for my OCD. I surround myself only with people I trust. And this is how I am able not to get lost and stuck in its web. I have found that there are three basic options for every single obsession and compulsion: to rebel, to avoid, or to obey. I spend most of my day rebelling and this is how I can stay productive.

Another way I have been able to beat the compulsions is through my religion. I realize that I am obeying a dictator if I listen to OCD's commands. Therefore, I cross myself and tell OCD that I am going to obey God's commandments and not OCD's, because He is my master and not OCD.

I have come to liken my experience of OCD to the way John Nash, the subject of the film *A Beautiful Mind*, experienced his schizophrenia. I still get the obsessions and the corresponding compulsions, just as he still saw people who weren't really there. However, like Nash, I know they are not real and I simply do not acknowledge them.

I am happy to report as the years go by, OCD does not and will not run my life as it once did. The guilt and shame and fear have receded into a distant memory, due to my constant disobedience. OCD will push hard with one of these compulsions daily, and I will have to battle it back. But once I do, it recedes and that is that. Only rarely do I catch myself obeying any of the compulsions

OCD springs on me. I have a great deal of trouble still with the pure obsessions but through recognizing them for what they are I am usually able not to allow them to take over.

OCD is a tyrant, a bully, a dictator. It is relentless and it is an almost impossible foe. However, I always remember that simple rule that I have written in my journals many times: I feed OCD by obedience and starve it by disobedience. This rule, and the knowledge that it really is powerless to do the things it threatens, can embolden almost anyone who fights this demon to make his or her life more bearable. It is anything but easy at first, but after you understand it, it becomes like the scenes at the end of *The Matrix*: you are in control. One can think of OCD as the bully we all knew in high school, the pseudo-tough guy who was, in reality, a coward—and you knew he was a coward because when you challenged him, he backed down.

I know that I will never destroy OCD and that it will always be in my head, shouting its commands. But I also know that it will never destroy me because I will fight back every step of the way with the support and tools I have acquired. OCD enslaved me and kept me enslaved until I got educated and fought back. Education, family support, and rebellion enabled and continue to enable me to stand up to the dictator in my head.

....

Kurt Warner has a bachelor's degree in English literature and a master's degree in social work. His work has been published in the academic journal Disability and Society, *and he has been a contributor to the newsletter of the Mental Health Association of Cortland County in New York.*

IN MINNESOTA, ONCE: ON ANOREXIA, MASCULINITY, AND RECOVERY

Owen Vince

For a year at the end of the Second World War, the American dietitian and scientist Ancel Keys led a long-term experiment at the University of Minnesota. Thirty-six volunteers, all of whom were conscientious objectors serving in Civilian Public Service (CPS) units, were guided through a program of controlled starvation and recovery. It is known today, simply, as the Minnesota Starvation Experiment. Keys's aim was to study the psychological and physiological effects of prolonged starvation, and to assess the process of rehabilitation. He had been, since the 1930s, interested in the militarization of food restriction; his research had led to the development of the so-called K-ration, a standard food pack supplied to soldiers serving overseas. Altogether, the experiment would aim to understand how best to rehabilitate famine victims and war refugees across Europe and Asia, to care and provide for those who had suffered not only emotionally but nutritionally. Its methods were new and quite startling: over a period of six months, thirty-six previously healthy male volunteers followed a strict reduction diet; in so doing, they lost considerable amounts of weight and also began to acquire new traits—apathy, short tempers, obsessive fascinations with food. As one participant later put it, "It made food the most important thing in one's life . . . food became the one central and only thing." For the first time, under scientific conditions, it was seen what happens to the mind as well as the body under conditions of immense restriction and control.

I first learned about what had happened in Minnesota when I was eighteen. Not from a history book, and not while idly thumbing through a newspaper or browsing a webpage. I was handed a small and largely uninformative pamphlet about the experiment by a well-meaning but apologetic nurse in the outpatient ward of a suburban mental health unit north of London. I was nearly sixty pounds underweight, with a BMI of about fifteen, and wanted—by hook or by crook—my life to end right there. I was suffering from the destructive patterns and behaviors of *anorexia nervosa*. I was also a young man. I suppose that explained her confusion. "We don't get any men with eating disorders," I was told.

I took that pamphlet away with me when I left the appointment, bundled up thickly in layers like I was Captain Scott heading out into the wintry dun of the Antarctic cold. I took it home and read about the men who had volunteered for Ancel Keys. I read about what had happened to them in those Minnesota dormitories; of how these ordinary, perhaps extraordinary, men, who had shunned the war for a variety of religious and moral reasons, who had been bullied and heckled for not being "real men," showed themselves, and maybe the world, that they *could* do violence—if only to themselves. That they could put their lives aside in order to save the lives of others.

What was compelling, in a dull and aching way, were not the details of the experiment itself—its clinical regulations, its aims, its measurements (though I memorized and studied these compulsively)—but the experiences of those thirty-six men. I read about how they, who had never shown signs of mental illness in their lives, grew neurotic, angry, obsessive. About how they grew thin. I recognized the same sad signs in myself. For over a month I had been receiving treatment at the ward, referred there by a concerned doctor. While I appreciated then—and still do, today— that they could have been the right people for some patients, I also recognized that what they were doing was something I could do myself, if I wanted to. The problem was both my assurance that the problem was *mine* to handle my way, and the realization that I didn't necessarily *want* things to change in the first place. I was eighteen, headstrong, probably a little arrogant. Perceiving what I saw as an intense femininity to the disease—not helped by its public perception—I adopted a dual tactic of both hiding it from the outside world and ignoring it. My efforts to withdraw myself from treatment were aided by reaching a certain designated target weight. Reach that, I thought, and they're off my back. It became a peculiar game of weights and balances, a sort of crooked game of chess. When you suffer from anorexia, you become very subtle. You have to. Eighteen *should* have been the age I went out into the world. I'd finished school and had places at universities, just a slow summer away. I'd made the decision a year earlier not to enter the army, which I recognize now as one of my better life decisions. I was healthy, athletic, and—for the most part—reasonably confident. And yet, I'd struggled with my weight as a child—being very tall meant that I had grown up quickly and put on some weight, which had become a nagging anxiety. I had also always been, in quiet little ways, quite obsessive, prone to form patterns out of otherwise patternless life. Throughout my younger years I had been less successful than I wanted to be at school, lonely, and acutely aware of my body as a thing that changed. Stopping short at eighteen, I imagine, something in my head—something small but load-bearing—had buckled under a mass of expectations, experiences, and self-judgments that culminated in my withdrawing from my friends (who began living *their* adult lives) and into myself.

It was around that time that my body stepped center stage. Something, in this weird life crisis, that I could definitely control. I knew *that* from past experience, from the shedding of teenage weight. I strapped on my trainers and hit the roads, quiet and breathless, at night. I began to put myself through a personal health revolution, convincing myself that it was about purifying my body, honing it. The problem was, I couldn't turn back from that. The less in control I felt about my life—my friends were away and I was living at home, with no idea what I wanted to do and only a kitchen job to show for my days, having decided on withdrawing from university—the more pressure I applied to the things over which I did have control. I ran farther. I ate less.

That pamphlet came at a good time. It was actually more useful, more important, than the nurse had perhaps realized. While I saw its limitations, I also saw it as a springboard to explore other possibilities—like recovery, like pulling myself out of this slick downward spiral in which I was caught. Because the volunteers had recovered, at least their weight, and had gone on to do impressive, worldly things, and to become interesting people, I saw an escape route. I imagined that if I could be *like them*, then there was a window through which I could escape it all. Recovery would become not simply about saving myself; rather, it would allow me to focus and pull myself into something else, something whole and positive. In a sense, I had seen what I was capable of—a furious and intense energy. All I needed, it seemed, confusingly, was to direct that energy to some other, better purpose. Of course, this was almost all I had to hold on to. I'd been offered treatment, but was agitated by its condescensions and the simple, awkward embarrassment of *being* in that situation—a situation that I had, it seemed, created for myself. I allowed my contact with the treatment center to die away, preferring instead my own path to recovery, feeling that it wasn't something that somebody could describe to me, but something that I'd simply alight on myself. For this, it was important to keep myself out of the hospital. Remaining in an outpatient ward allowed me that little freedom to make my own choices, my own decisions. In a sense, it was my mind pressing down hard on the brake pedal. Recovery became something intimately personal, a path I gleaned from what I thought I knew about myself. I labored under the—perhaps delusional— idea that when the time was right, I could simply flick a switch and return to something approaching an ordinary life.

But that sense of being "in control" came only on a good day. One of the characteristic compulsions of my disorder was not simply to restrict my food in crushing details—so that the often banal, usually enjoyable experience of simply eating was blown up in all its proportions into a monotonous form of hard labor—but to have a constant, abstracted urge to maintain precisely this activity. It manifested into a kind of fear of food—or, not food *as such*, but the possibility of losing minute control over food. There was no fear attached to what I had *allowed* myself to consume, but there was to all food outside of that. It was, at its core, a fear of the loss of control. And, eating being an act of control, the food became a lever—something that diminished each day as I pressed harder on it. If eating was control, then to eat *less* food conferred greater control. It was a familiar, albeit inane, feat of engineering. There was little rationality attached to this, except my own. And, like anyone under siege, I adopted the siege mentality—everything *out there* was somehow wrong, while what I was doing (defending myself!) was naturally and inviolably *correct*. This mentality contributes to that sense of dysmorphia—but despite their fixation on imagined or minor defects, anorexia sufferers believe that they are fine and actually very much "in control." In reality, they spin out of control. That tremulous line between the real and our perception of it becomes entirely destructed.

As a result of this, I shivered at the thought of deviation from what I had "allowed" myself to do, to eat. In my life, I have never been more controlled, dedicated, determined—it is just a shame that that energy, the little I had, was being committed to such self-destructive ends. For me, several memories stand out from that time—some of them are physical, sensations. Others are impressions. I remember being tired—eternally tired, the feeling of being drained right down to the marrow of my bones. I remember being cold, regardless of the room's temperature, the weather. Everything is cast in this endless, furtive winter. I became solitary. I remember withdrawal. I remember my memory itself unwinding. I struggled to concentrate on things—words, ideas, conversation. When you turn in toward your self, your body, in its mental frostbite, sheds what is unnecessary. Some nights I struggled to sleep. Some days I couldn't pull myself out of bed. Everything—everything with which I came into contact—soured me, scraped against me. Your body becomes more sensitive, frailer. And you are trapped there, in a slowly, slowly shrinking room. The lights flicker.

In that thick fug, I couldn't perceive the strain it put on the people close to me, who saw this once healthy, handsome young man become a sort of shell, a skeleton. It's like I was becoming transparent, fading from this life and heading for some other, sad shore. I had intolerable arguments with my family, and closed down any close relationships with friends. I was proud and bitter. I wanted them to reassure me that I was thin, thinner. It brought me comfort. A sort of logic. But I was also ashamed. I was like a wounded creature.

A moving and meaningful article in the *Guardian* by another male sufferer once described this as the "secret world of male anorexia." A secret, a cloying and clotted embarrassment. Because the media so readily paint self-starvation as a solely feminine experience—I don't know whether out of ignorance or conceit—as the "holy anorexia," the "beauty queen" body obsession (and other unfair clichés for those women and girls who also suffer), male sufferers are caught in the position of anxious, awkward impossibility. Not only do we have to cope with the illness, we also have to cope with the incomprehension of those who do not believe we should have it in the first place. I *knew* there were other male sufferers. I never felt like contacting them in my lone wolf therapy, but I knew I could not be, was not, alone in this. And yet, the sensitivity to the world of representations is endless; representations of "the male," of male beauty, of manliness, have the same contours and effects as those of the feminine. In magazines, men are stubble-faced, thick-shouldered, confident. Or else models, who are tall and wiry and sharp-faced. Even now, mirrors are not just reflectors but traps—places in which my body is presented to me. I am ever cautious and aware of tracking the changes that have occurred on it. When I first entered the spiral of reduced eating and overexercising—and how strange it must have seemed when in restaurants the young, thin man ordered the meal without cheese, asked if they could leave out the mayonnaise, asked if they had diet drinks—it was a process continuously checked by worldly perceptions and reactions. When I was the runner ruining myself over hard-won miles, along roads and tracks and paths, an old teacher commenting on my loss of weight, even a little concern edging her voice, was a "good" thing. The people who said, "You look different," were inviting a sharp possibility— *different*. "Thicker or thinner?" my curiosity drove me to ask. I implored friends to delete photos of me from their Facebook pages—"Why?" "Just do it. It doesn't make any difference to you. I just don't like it." A lot of these people I haven't spoken to since. It was easier to spend time alone, because in public— around people—there was the possibility that they would say the slightest, most meaningless thing, and it would be picked apart by me. A throwaway comment, like—because I've always been tall with big shoulders, but carried some puppy fat as a teenager—"big guy," or when people said, "You're a size thirty-four, right?" When the man in the shop, from whom I was buying a small-sized shirt, said, "You sure? Not medium?" To them, a saying they'll forget, while for me these became ingrained and fatal remarks. I was as sensitive to language as a translator, as a linguist. I even remember, once, shivering in thick clothes as I walked through a deserted shopping center in the early morning, how two people passed and one of them laughed, said something. It sounded like "fat." It couldn't have been—they weren't even looking at me. I was about 105 pounds. But to my poisoned mind, they had called me fat. I didn't eat for about two days. Men, too, are expected to be certain ways. How they look, act, and think. Manliness is a physical imagination, even in its social aspects—men are "forthright," decisive, leaders. But when we *break* those expectations, whether voluntarily or not, it becomes very hard to claw our way back to "normality"—in my case, rehabilitation—without reference *to* that masculinity. My recovery had to be strong, lone, and decisive. I still don't know what to make of this. I at least worry less, now, about manly expectations. I've spent my time writing poetry, but also digging holes in the earth under the high, bright sun. I think—now—I see a balance.

• • •

My grandmother was dying. From dementia. She was—in an echo of myself—fading away from us. A buildup of plaque on the brain, a distortion and erosion of who she once was. She shrunk into nothing, while my grandfather sat beside her with endlessly patient and sorrowful eyes, feeding her spoonfuls of food as if she were a child. Food that she spat at him, or let fall from her mouth.

Her death, during my illness, formed a strong influence on me. Where she had no control over what was happening to her, and while it felt like I too had none, I knew that wasn't true. I understood in that glimpsed reflection of myself, that what I was doing was destructive, inane. That it was stupid.

One of the uncomfortable facts of excavating this past is the strange effect that it had on my inner timeline. It's as if all of that experience—for that year unlike no other—has become compressed, distorted. Trying accurately to pinpoint one thing and its temporal relationship to another is hard. This fracture-world of memories is the legacy of what happened to me. The way you can see a flood's devastation of a landscape long after the waters have receded.

For me, on the path to recovery, it was essential not only to take control (a different kind of control, a positive control, which was actually a form of letting go) of my condition, but to locate my experience outside of myself. Not to abstract it, but to locate it personally, emotionally in other people and experiences. For the worst six months of my illness, when I was threatened with being sectioned under the Mental Health Act and force-fed for my own well-being, I was locked in to myself, focusing everything inward—where all this energy met in the surface and meat of my body. If I couldn't tear out and remake my heart and brain, I could remake my body; I could control it and hammer it. Exhaustion and weightlessness were for me the keys and signs that I was narrowing to a point, eclipsing myself. It was necessary for me, by inches, by pounds, to narrow down this existence—

when I weighed 150 pounds, and then 140, and then 130. When my BMI crept down by 0.1, by 0.2, by a whole point. When on the charts I slipped from green to red. I knew these were abstractions, guides—but I had to match up to them. It was a senseless, numbing arithmetic.

I began to direct the energies and obsessions of controlling my food toward the kinds of ethical responsibilities that Keys's volunteers had achieved. It was almost a form of pretend, an imagination or delusion, but the idea was sure and secure; it excused me of the thing about which I was most shocked and embarrassed, that I was a man, undergoing an experience—as I was told again and again—that men "didn't get." I knew that was incorrect—I know the statistics: three in one thousand men are supposed to suffer from an eating disorder. But it was depressing and alienating to read leaflets and advice about anorexia when the only personal pronouns used were *her* or *she*, the only references to teenage girls. There was no *he*, no *him*. No grown men. But there were Keys's volunteers. I don't know how useful it is to talk about "male anorexia"—qualitatively, each sufferer is unique. The mechanics may be the same (starvation, obsessive exercise, and so on), but the inner world is distinct. I can't help but reach back to my childhood for the root of all this. From birth, I was quite a "sickly" child—asthma, eczema, and lactose intolerance. I managed to shrug these off for the most part when we moved from the city to the countryside—the clearer air purging my lungs. I did a *lot* of sport—football, cricket, swimming. Almost every day I was muddying myself in fields and pushing against my body's retaliation, the tightness in my chest. Despite this, I was always behind the boys my age—never fast enough, never quite keeping up. I exhausted myself in this. From this, I idealized what I wanted to be—fit, strong, and exceptional. Simply trying hard wasn't enough for me. It never has been, when it comes down to my body. At that age I learned the ways in which the body responded to what you *did* to it—my bigness was an issue, because it slowed me down. Less food meant a faster body. A better sportsman. Punishing myself on rain-wet football fields meant that I learned harder, would prove myself. I broke my hand twice doing this, and would sometimes return home so hammered by the effort that I would spend the night strapped into an inhaler, struggling out every breath. I have always seen the effort of pushing the body to be a somehow *heroic* thing, a thing that is not simply a "hobby" or "something you do," but an expected thing that "men" *must do*. I read up on the early Olympic games, of Greek men who ran, fought, struggled to make themselves into the beautiful idea of the athlete warrior. My fascination with archaeology stemmed from the pageantry and heroic ideal of this athlete, in my imaginings of what Paul Treherne, writing in the *European Journal of Archaeology*, has called "an equally distinctive notion of male *beauty*, unique to the warrior," a beauty that manifested itself in the preparation of the body, in its comportment and action in running, struggling, acting. This was precisely the anachronistic and ill-fitting ideal that I tried to force my life into and around. And yet, its outcome was something else—a humiliating denial of that same masculinity, its reduction and destruction. I wonder, even now, if somehow subconsciously I had set myself on this path in order to free myself of something poisonous.

And so, there was a sense, a feeling, that my anorexia was linked intrinsically to ideas I held about masculinity, about the male body, about sex and sexuality. That I was trying to *prove* something. But recovery was also about proving something, a way of justifying what I had done to myself without having to acknowledge that I had failed those ideals that had sustained me for so long. I had to locate my recovery personally in an ethical act that went beyond this *thing* that I was doing to myself. Just, perhaps, as the volunteers in Minnesota had proved that they could suffer and feel fear and pain just like soldiers, but for the good of others, for civilian and scientific reasons. This, at least, was my narrative—the narrative that pulled me out of it. It placed the experience within a familiar—and, importantly, a masculine—frame of reference that gave me the impression of doing something strong and willful; it was no longer "feminine," humiliating, because others had done this thing, and had done it in an ethically responsible, masculine way. It was like I had socialized my recovery, turning it into an invisible civic good that would result, as it had with the conscientious objectors, as something that I had *gone through* with honor and strength, without sliding into what I saw at the time—unfairly—as a weakness. I was hard on myself. Harder still on other sufferers, whom I shunned the idea of. It was a recovery. But a patchwork recovery. It had arrogance and not a little coldness.

Anorexia, for me, was a denial of at least the idea of masculinity. But before it got to its worst, when it had worked its way into my core, I had been like a "normal" young man: sex drive, girlfriends, football, and parties. I was always thoughtful, introverted, bookish, but in a balanced way in which I could at least give the impression of living outside of myself. Anorexia, in fact any eating disorder, has always been imagined as a feminine issue. That it is about "body image" and the misrepresentations of femininity in popular media. Body image has a great deal to do with anorexia and bulimia, but that is—as any sufferer will tell you—not the whole story. Body image is a hook, a mechanism of reduction, of closing down the self. It is the logical extension of *wiping out* your self from the world, from the external, uncontrollable world, without having to take the step of killing yourself. For me, reducing my body was the equivalent of disappearing while still keeping a foothold in the world. Harold Blickenstaff, one of the Minnesota project's volunteers, explained this strange estrangement from normality like this, that "I had just decided that this was what I was going to do and so I was going to do it . . . and so I would say walking by a bakery was like walking by a bank. It might be nice to have what's in there, but it's out of the question. I never debated whether or not I should break diet or do anything else." It was a dedication beyond reason, beyond what was "good" for me or "bad." It was a cycle, a dependency. It was just like that, except I hadn't decided anything.

Unlike Keys's volunteers, I had no mandated reason for my starvation. I wasn't the volunteer in an experiment. I had taken this route by myself, out of some hazy constellation of urges and ideas and difficulties. I had to map out the period in my mind, tracing it back perhaps to the awkward surge of my growth when I was a young teenager (towering weirdly above my classmates). Or perhaps to my sicknesses as a child; to the eczema and asthma which crippled me in a hospital for the first year of my life. Perhaps it was also the cognitive dissonance of the difficulties involved in securing my introverted, sensitive inner self from the social, heady adult world into which I was pitched. It was the recognition of my failures, that I had struggled academically at school despite my talents and energies and insights. And I had always had few friends, but many "sort of" friends. Lots of people to party and mess about with, yet very few on whom to unburden myself. Perhaps it was a combination of all of these things. Perhaps there was no single "trigger." And yet, I saw in Keys's volunteers the same thoughts that I'd had. Faced with accusations of cowardice and "not being men," by refusing to fight they did something equally harmful and dangerous, proving that they could do violence, that they could have an almost inhuman strength. Some CPS volunteers "smoke jumped," parachuting near forest fires to tackle the blaze. Others built roads, worked in mines, felled trees. And some starved. Willingly, they starved and recovered themselves, tipping at the brink. It's as if I had decided I was *one of them*, the thirty-seventh volunteer. That my illness—and its recovery— had some fulfilling, dangerous purpose by which I could justify it, through which I could make it seem not like a personal failure, but a personal victory, a badge of honor, giving rather than taking; that I clove and fought through to my own recovery—a singular act, a pressure of will—was necessary because of the root of the problem itself, that masculine self-reliance that fueled my self-destruction. The only way out meant going back to the source, excavating down to the roots—ripping them out of the soil.

That I can write this essay at all is a positive sign. It is the acknowledgement that I underwent that experience, and pulled myself out of it. For many years afterward, while at university where I relapsed and ended up in the strange medium ground of bulimia nervosa, I was unable to acknowledge that part or aspect of my life. I shut it away, locked the door, threw away the key (and other worn metaphors). I destroyed all reference to it—medical documents, appointment cards, writings, scribbles, e-mails. I hid associative objects away—photographs, purchases, clothes. Burying it was a dangerous ploy, I knew, just a form of avoidance. Part of the motion of recovery is not simply to recover, I think, but to accept the illness as part of you. Easier said than done, of course, as always. And recovery, I know, is a process—an ongoing and everlasting thing. It is not an event, an act; it is a shift in perception and living. An important part of that was learning not to expect so much of myself. That, by projecting myself onto some arcane ideal, I was simply chasing smoke rather than getting at the very personal, subjective reasons of why I unraveled when I did.

And so, writing this—writing about my Minnesota—is a part of that. A locating of my illness in the world around me, but also an acknowledgement, an acceptance. Perhaps, if you were feeling generous, you would say that I had taken responsibility for it. I think that part of that responsibility stemmed from the knowing that if I were to allow myself to fade away, I would no longer have a grasp on the beautiful and wavering things of this world; even now, when I feel sick and tired and my brain tries to claw inexpertly back to that former life, I think about the beautiful things that this healthy, living me can touch and hold on to. The fresh, fast sea breeze as it soars over the cliffs where I live, the paths and mud-thick fields and hills over which I run in spattered clothing and clawed running shoes; the taste of thick, bitter coffee on a winter morning; the smell of woodsmoke in the fireplace; the lulling, slow, luxurious words of W. G. Sebald, the animal sensuousness of Ted Hughes, the velveteen and quixotic marvel of Nabokov.

For me, these are sensual, as well as narrative, means to remain whole and healthy. I remind myself that the illusion of control that I drew from my anorexic suffering was really, truly a denial, a closing of the blinds, a strangling of self. It was only the impression of control. But, I learned, life isn't about control at all—not *real* life. Real life is vivid and unknown; it is about not shrinking to a point but expanding openly, unknowingly, into uncertainty. I know that now. I live that now. There's so much time to make up for, since I left the state to which I have never been—once I left Minnesota behind me.

....

Owen Vince is a poet and ambient music journalist living in rural west Wales. An archaeologist by trade, his work is heavily influenced by history, memory, and place, and has appeared in Magma, Aethlon, Butcher's Dog, *and* Cadaverine Magazine, *among others. He coedits a poetry magazine,* HARK, *and runs up mountains for sport.*

JEANNIE

Miriam Mandel Levi

Upon hearing the pleas of a desperate mother, a speech therapist agrees to take on an unusual patient. How can she help a young girl who has no apparent physical difficulties but simply chooses not to speak?

When unrestrained, Jeannie swallowed bolts and pencils, smashed her head against the floor, and tore strips of flesh from her arms with her teeth. "Like a Rottweiler," the charge nurse, Meg, said in our initial phone conversation. Jeannie had also slammed a doctor's head into a wall, causing a concussion. "But she has two full-time guards now," Meg assured me. They had been privately hired by Jeannie's parents at the insistence of the hospital administration.

The day after I spoke to Meg, I drove to the psychiatric facility where Jeannie was hospitalized. It was a warm spring day as I climbed the metal stairwell from the garden to the adolescent ward. The stairs were encased by a protective cage. Suicide prevention, I thought grimly. I pressed the intercom bell.

"She's waiting for you," Meg said in a hoarse smoker's voice when she came to the door. Her work boots clopped on the linoleum floor, and a large ring of keys jangled from a belt loop on her jeans. We walked down a long corridor.

"I'd like to take a look at her medical chart before I see her," I said.

Meg stopped and leaned back. She bent one knee and fixed the sole of her boot to the wall. "Ask me what you want to know," she said. Her eyes followed a lanky teenage boy who zigzagged by.

There was a toughness and resoluteness about Meg. She was letting me know, in no uncertain terms, that I was on her turf and playing by her rules. I didn't like that she denied me access to the medical chart, but I had the good sense to realize that if I wanted to make inroads with Jeannie, I had to ally myself with Meg. I took a pen and paper out of my briefcase and asked my questions.

Jeannie was eighteen years old. From the age of twelve, she had been in psychiatric institutions, diagnosed successively with depression, anorexia, personality disorder, and pervasive refusal syndrome. From one day to the next, Jeannie had stopped walking, eating, and speaking. A nasogastric tube had been inserted from her nose to her stomach to provide nourishment. Her hands had been tied to the iron grates of her bed to prevent her from yanking it out. Month after month, she had languished, wanting to die.

Yet, prior to my arrival, Jeannie had showed some signs of recovery. Although she could no longer walk due to muscle disuse, she had begun to crawl and was awaiting surgery to correct the damage her immobility had wrought. She had also begun to eat. "A raisin. That's what she agreed to eat the first day," Meg said, nodding in recollection. When Jeannie was eating enough calories, the nasogastric tube was removed. As the violence subsided, so did the use of restraints, which were currently applied only at night.

The staff's best efforts, however, had not succeeded in getting Jeannie to speak. She nodded yes and no and wrote messages on her phone but, apart from shrieking in protest, did not verbalize. For this reason, I had been asked to do a speech evaluation by Jeannie's mother, Katherine.

Keys clanged and locks clicked somewhere down the corridor. Behind a closed door, I heard sounds of a scuffle. As Meg and I approached the room, Jeannie peeked around the doorframe. I froze. She was on her hands and knees, her shoulders tense. Her hair, tangled and greasy, was pulled back in a ponytail. She watched me for several seconds with a fierce vigilance and then withdrew. I followed Meg tentatively into her room.

On the right was an iron-framed bed. From each corner hung a leather restraint. Over the bed was a worn world map. Straight ahead on the windowsill were assorted mementos—Russian nesting dolls, wooden shoes, a bronze dragon, and a snow globe. The window was barred. Jeannie's mother, a geneticist who traveled extensively for her work, brought the world back in bits for Jeannie.

Jeannie huddled on her bed and Meg flopped next to her. Two burly female guards in civilian dress slouched at the doorway. I introduced myself.

"I'm a speech language pathologist. I help people who have difficulty speaking. I'd like to see if I can help you, Jeannie."

I pulled a chair to the edge of the bed.

Jeannie was so thin I could see her bones. Her T-shirt and sweatpants drooped on her form. Her dark eyes would not settle on mine; they scuttled like insects to the corners of the room. She looked so fragile; it was hard to imagine her causing anyone harm. Nonetheless, I could feel the blood pulsing in my neck. I put on my best professional air and began the evaluation.

"Are you having difficulty speaking?"

Jeannie shrugged one shoulder.

"Can you tell me what the problem is?"

Jeannie rolled her eyes and looked at Meg.

"Don't ask me," Meg said, tossing Jeannie her phone.

Jeannie typed a message and held the screen up for Meg to read.

"She says she can't talk and you won't be able to help her."

I should have expected it, but her proclamation caught me off guard. The patients in my clinic wanted to get better. They were motivated, cooperative, and worked diligently in therapy. Jeannie, on the other hand, was thwarting me at the outset. We were off to a bad start. Meg's brusque manner seemed to get through to Jeannie, but that was not my style.

"Open your mouth wide . . . purse your lips, then retract them . . . stick out your tongue and press against this stick," I said.

"Do it, Jeannie," Meg ordered.

She had good movement of her jaw, lips, and tongue, certainly sufficient for producing speech. I asked her to cough and clear her throat, which she did, indicating that her vocal folds moved well and that she had the potential to produce a voice. Based on her case history and good oral motor skills, I concluded she had the physical ability to speak and was choosing not to, a condition called psychogenic mutism.

After the evaluation, Meg and I joined Jeannie's mother in the meeting room. It was a small room, windowless and dimly lit. Katherine looked to be in her forties, petite, with chin-length, wavy dark hair and a small mouth. She was dressed in neat, professional attire, charcoal pants and a collared blouse. But there was a woundedness about her. Her eyes were black and deep. She wrung her hands in her lap.

I explained the results of my assessment.

"I think it's a psychogenic, not an organic, speech problem. It needs to be treated by a psychiatrist, not by me. I can't help—I'm sorry."

I wasn't sorry though. I didn't want to take the case. Jeannie didn't want to speak, and she didn't want my help. There was no way I'd overcome her intransigence.

Katherine's face fell. "Please," she said, "nobody has been able to help. She's been treated by every psychiatrist and psychologist on staff. She's had private consultations. She won't speak. Try to understand—she hasn't said a word in six years."

The room was stifling. I loosened the scarf around my neck.

"It's outside my area of expertise," I replied. "I've never treated this kind of problem."

In general, I worked with adults who had neurologically based communication disorders. Over the years, I had treated cases of mutism due to profound language or neuromuscular impairment, but Jeannie's condition was different. She had no neurological history. Her CT scan and MRI were normal. She was choosing not to speak, and I didn't have the tools to help her.

Katherine suggested a short trial of therapy—five sessions. I sighed and told her I'd think about it. "I hope you'll agree," Katherine said, reaching out her hand. Our eyes met, and something inside me softened to her, for her love of this child and her enduring hope for a recovery. I knew I would say yes. I was a mother, too.

At home, I researched pervasive refusal syndrome (PRS). A newly described and contested disorder, it was documented for the first time just over twenty years ago. PRS is most commonly seen in girls between the ages of eight and fifteen. As in Jeannie's case, sufferers withdraw socially and refuse to eat, drink, talk, walk, or engage in any kind of self-care. In most cases, patients experience a deep sense of helplessness and hopelessness. PRS shares many features with other psychiatric diagnoses like depression, anorexia, and catatonic and conversion disorders. For that reason, its detractors do not view it as a separate entity. Proponents, on the other hand, claim that it is distinct from the other disorders in its sufferers' active resistance to any form of help. PRS is not included in the *Diagnostic and Statistical Manual of Mental Disorders* and seems more widely accepted in the European than the North American psychiatric community. The mainstays of treatment are patience, time, basic nursing care, physiotherapy, and counseling.

I found no information on speech therapy for this condition. Perhaps the treatments were not documented or patients spontaneously regained their speech when they were ready. But for Jeannie, it had been six years.

One week later I returned to the facility with a plan. I would begin by teaching Jeannie the mechanics of speech. Meg had told me that she was intelligent and curious; this approach might make her more of a partner in the therapy process. I came with diagrams, explanations, and video clips of vocal folds vibrating. We reviewed the basics of respiration, phonation, resonance, and articulation. Jeannie followed closely, then, with hand signals, indicated that I should send her the URL of the vocal folds clip so she could watch it on her phone. I was encouraged.

Therapies for communication disorders are often most effective when administered several times a week. However, I decided to treat Jeannie once a week. Recovery in PRS is slow; too aggressive a course of treatment can result in relapse. The person with PRS may perceive the rehabilitation as coercive, feel more helpless, and regress. Although I suspected Jeannie had the full ability to speak, I would treat her the same as any patient with a severe motor speech disorder. We would progress vowel by vowel, consonant by consonant, from syllables to words to sentences. Meg offered to attend the sessions. Her presence reassured Jeannie and ensured her cooperation.

The following week, I began to work with the one feature of speech Jeannie had—a voice. Although she used her voice only to grunt or screech, we would shape the sound into something meaningful. I checked to make sure she could identify how many syllables were in a word. Jeannie sat on the edge of her bed, hands in her lap. Meg sat next to Jeannie, her back to the wall, legs splayed, texting on her phone. I leaned forward in my chair.

"Make a sound," I said.

"Uh," she responded.

"Now make two."

She looked at me suspiciously. "Uh uh."

So it went for three and four and five sounds. I then used the vocalizations in a game. Meg had told me that Jeannie liked geography and knew the names of every country and capital city. I would tell her the name of a country and she would tell me the name of the capital city, the correct number of grunts for the syllables in the word.

When Jeannie saw the direction of the task, she raised her upper lip in a snarl, then slammed the wall with the back of her hand and screeched. She thought I was tricking her to use her voice for communication and she was mad. I didn't anticipate the hostile outburst but reacted quickly, pushing my chair back out of her reach. The guards stepped forward.

Meg grabbed her wrist. "If you want your privileges today, cooperate." Jeannie quieted and glared at me. I stared back and resumed the task.

"Canada," I said, steadying my voice.

"Uh-uh-uh," she said with a sneer.

"Right, Ottawa," I replied. "Here's a hard one—Uruguay."

Jeannie eyed me. She didn't want to answer but the challenge was irresistible.

"Uh-uh-uh-uh-uh."

"Montevideo. Good for you," I said, smiling.

One of the guards said, "Yeah, Jeannie." Jeannie shrieked again, narrowed her eyes, and tensed her muscles as if to pounce. Then she swiveled on the bed and turned her back to me. The session was over, but I was satisfied we had achieved meaningful, if rudimentary, communication.

Later I learned enthusiastic reactions are almost always counterproductive in PRS. Jeannie had probably perceived my positivity as a celebration of victory over her resistance. I would have to unlearn ingrained positive responses. Rehabilitation professionals like me are the cheerleaders of the medical world. Our mottoes are hope and progress. Jeannie's were hopelessness and resistance.

If the first two sessions gave me hope for Jeannie's recovery, the next three were discouraging. Jeannie would do anything with her articulators—purse her lips, lift her tongue tip to her palate—as long as it wasn't paired with voice for speech. When she sensed I was moving her toward sound production, even a simple vowel, she shut down. Three weeks passed without progress, and our five agreed-upon sessions were over.

I wasn't surprised she hadn't responded to my methods. I wasn't the right professional to treat her and shouldn't have let myself be persuaded. I would tell Katherine by e-mail that I was terminating therapy.

Dear Katherine,

I have completed five sessions with Jeannie. However, she does not seem to be responding to my interventions.

I bowed my head and pressed my eyelids. When I looked up the words on the screen had blurred.

Perhaps we can take advantage of Jeannie's texting. There is an application for smartphones that translates written text to oral speech. She could type and the phone would "speak" her message.

It was such an inadequate solution. I immediately deleted what I had written.

I'm sure there is another professional more qualified to help her.

Was there? An army of professionals had already tried. Still, there was always the possibility, however unlikely, that Jeannie would resume speaking of her own accord.

I am truly sorry and wish the best for—

I thought of my own children, then of Katherine. I saw her petite form hunched over the computer, her eyes dark wells, her hope for Jeannie so nearly drained. I began again:

Our five sessions are up, but I think Jeannie needs more time. If it's okay with you, I'd like to do another round of five sessions.

The following week we began round two. Jeannie disrupted the sessions by checking the time on her phone and by pulling the skin on her stomach to gauge her body fat. I told her that if she worked undistracted for twelve minutes, she would earn a three-minute break. During the breaks, we would read *Ripley's Believe It or Not!*

Jeannie loved *Ripley's*. She was fascinated by the girl who sweated blood, the boy with eight toes on each foot, the man with a hole in his chin, held agape by a transparent disc. While this sorry parade of humanity revolted me, it delighted Jeannie. Maybe she felt an affinity to these deviant folk. Maybe she saw them as archetypes of a cruel, absurd world.

I worked painstakingly over the subsequent weeks to elicit a vowel sound from Jeannie. I explained how vowels are formed by varying lip position and tongue and jaw height. With diagrams, mirrors, and modeling, I shaped the correct mouth posture for each vowel. One day, I finally asked her to add a voice and say the vowel aloud.

Jeannie was suddenly concerned. She tapped Meg's arm and wrote a word in the air with her index finger.

"Progress?" Meg said. "You think that if you learn to make the vowel sound, you'll be progressing?" Her sarcasm was intentional. If Jeannie sensed we were taking steps toward improvement, she would stop cooperating. Meg went on. "Asking me how I'm feeling today would be progress," she said. Meg spoke Jeannie's language of derision. But she was devoted to her and Jeannie knew it.

"Jeannie," I said, "you have a voice and you have the correct mouth position. Put them together. There is no reason you can't do it."

Jeannie screwed up her face in a show of effort and emitted a series of coughs.

"No. Try again. Round your lips. Now make a sound."

She rounded her lips and made some guttural noises. I gritted my teeth. Meg shot her a threatening look.

"O," Jeannie croaked.

I startled. Meg looked up from her phone. Even the guards turned their heads. Jeannie watched our reactions intently. A few seconds of silence elapsed, then Meg said: "What do you expect? That we're going to jump up and down because you made a sound? Big deal, Jeannie."

I bit my lip to suppress a smile and, taking my cue from Meg, moved on, casually, to the next task.

Our indifferent responses told Jeannie it was safe to proceed, that she hadn't made any movement toward recovery or life. It was important she believe she had done nothing to excite or please us. Otherwise she would undo the little progress she had made. In the next session, *o* led to *e,* and the rest of the vowels and consonants followed. I sent Katherine an update.

Jeannie is making progress. She is saying individual sounds.

I was beginning to believe that traditional speech therapy was the right prescription for Jeannie's problem after all. She needed a process that was gradual enough that she felt in control.

The threat of sanctions helped too. The chief psychiatrist had told her that if she wanted to remain on the unit, she had to participate in rehabilitative efforts. When Jeannie was being particularly contrary, Meg reminded her that she could lose an hour in the TV or Snoezelen multisensory rooms. In the soothing Snoezelen room, Jeannie enjoyed a variety of sights, sounds, movements, textures, and smells, all of which she controlled. It was her favorite time of the day.

If our first hurdle had been the production of a recognizable sound, the next was the production of a word. I knew this transition would be difficult for Jeannie. Isolated sounds carried no meaning, but a word had communicative value.

I entered the psychiatric ward to the usual jangling of keys and clanging of locks. A teenage girl greeted me singing one line from *The Sound of Music* over and over: "When the dog bites, when the bee stings." A boy with pimples stood facing a wall, snickering. I walked into Jeannie's room and gasped. Running down the side of her neck were three deep red and purple gashes. When Jeannie saw my expression of horror, she smiled. Meg told me that she had lacerated her neck with a sharp stone she'd found on the hospital grounds. I felt sick for her tortured self.

Even if Jeannie were to regain speech, to what purpose would she use it? When her family members visited, she spit and clawed at them. Success in speech therapy might simply translate those behaviors to insults and curses.

I teach my students who are studying to become speech language pathologists that communication interaction can be divided into four functional categories: expression of basic wants and needs, information transfer, social closeness, and social etiquette. I could imagine the day Jeannie would use spoken language to meet her basic needs—to request a drink or a sweater, even eventually to exchange ideas. But social closeness was unimaginable. I looked at her mutilated neck and her ghoulish grin. It was hard to believe that, even with the ability to speak, she would ever break out of her dark torment to form a close bond with another person.

Jeannie resisted saying a word. She inserted a pause in the middle and broke the word into its constituent sounds. She produced the word with an inaudible voice or with minimal movements of her lips and tongue to render it unintelligible. We tried again and again to blend the component sounds together, to raise the volume of her voice, to exaggerate the movements of her mouth. As the sessions passed, my hope waned. I dreaded telling Katherine our venture had failed. I had one last idea—the word *no*. It was Jeannie's rallying cry, the word she would most want to say. I pulled my chair closer to the edge of the bed until my knees and Jeannie's were touching.

"Say no."

"N . . . o."

"Put the sounds together like this: no." I pronounced the word slowly and clearly.

"Mmmm."

"Come on," I said. "You know that's not the right sound."

I could hear the rebuke in my voice. My well-practiced patience was wearing thin. I softened my tone and began again.

"Put your tongue behind your front teeth for *n* and round your lips for *o*."

"Mmm."

"No," I said.

"N."

I banged the arms of my chair with the palms of my hands. "Jeannie—it's not that difficult."

She sat up straight, cocked her head, then motioned to Meg to send the guards out of the room. I threw Meg an imploring glance. I wanted Jeannie to say her first word as much as anyone but not at the risk of my safety. Meg met my gaze and nodded reassuringly. The guards lumbered out of the room and closed the door behind them.

I nudged my chair back out of Jeannie's reach, and we resumed where we'd left off. I took a deep breath.

"Again, Jeannie, say no. Both sounds together."

"N."

"Watch me and do what I do—no."

"O."

"Both sounds. Look in the mirror with me."

"N . . . o."

"Without a pause in the middle."

"Uh," she said with facial contortions for added effect.

"Stop playing games." If I didn't hear a word today, I wasn't coming back. Four months of therapy and I hadn't extracted a single word from her. It was hopeless.

"M," she said.

"No."

"O."

"Say it," I said.

Jeannie gasped, "No."

There it was, so long awaited, so weighty it seemed to assume a corporeal form. We shifted in our chairs, uneasy in the presence of its strange company. Jeannie folded at the waist and tucked her head between her knees, in a posture of submission or relief or both. Meg and I looked at each other in bewilderment. I was worn out and hopeful. Perhaps at the end of this long, arduous process, Jeannie would finally speak.

The following session, Jeannie said *yes* and we played a game in which she picked a country, and I had to guess her choice by asking twenty yes/no questions. She chose obscure countries like Guernsey and Comoros and mocked me when I didn't guess them, but I took the defeat in stride; my victory was her responses.

Though she had progressed, Jeannie's speech was far from normal. Her voice was croaked and dry, like something long buried and unearthed. It resonated in her nose with a muffled quality and made her sound as if she were ailing or dying. As long as I could decipher the word, I didn't care. I knew she needed to keep up the fight.

Several sessions passed in which we expanded Jeannie's vocabulary. I said a word, and she produced an antonym or synonym, or she guessed a word that I defined. In another task, I presented faces of famous people and had her name them—Jesus, Napoleon, the Beatles. She even identified J. K. Rowling and Steve Jobs. The tasks challenged and entertained Jeannie and, moreover, distracted her from the fact that she was speaking. Within a few weeks, we advanced to sentences.

One day, as I showed Jeannie pictures to describe, she clamped down and refused to talk about an ice cream cone. Meg cracked a smile. "There are too many calories in the ice cream. She might gain weight if she describes it."

Jeannie's lips pulled back to reveal small, eroded teeth. She inhaled jaggedly, then choked out a laugh. Meg fell over on the bed snorting. I threw my head back and laughed. At that moment, I half believed Jeannie would declare the show was over, that she was done with the mental illness. We could all pack up and go home.

I told Jeannie we had one final goal. She had to use the words she had mastered in therapy on the ward. She whispered something to Meg.

"Laugh at you? You're crawling on the floor and squawking and you're not worried anyone's going to find that strange. But if you say a word, people are going to laugh?"

Jeannie bit her nails. In some strange way, she cared what others thought of her. Hearing her express such normal adolescent insecurity made me want to hug and reassure her. Somewhere along the way, I had developed an affection for Jeannie, for her frightened, frightful soul.

As her first word outside therapy, Jeannie chose *awful* in order to answer people when they asked how she was feeling. The following week she chose *yes* and *no*. We posted a list of the words on her wall to enlist the staff in encouraging their use. The plan was to add one or two new words each week.

"At this rate, you'll be speaking fluently by the time you're eighty," Meg said.

That night Katherine wrote me.

Miriam,

I spoke to Jeannie on the phone tonight and she answered yes and no to my questions. I can't tell you how emotional it was for me to hear her speak again after so many years. I am so grateful to you for all you have done.

Five months had passed since we began treatment. Though she continued to use a gravelly voice and was frugal with her words, Jeannie spoke in full sentences in therapy and was using some twenty words and phrases on the ward. These included basic requests like *bathroom* and *medication* as well as *How many calories?* and *Leave me alone*. She refused to say *Mom* or *Meg*, *hello* or *thank you*.

I suspected that with time, Jeannie would get used to her speaking self, expand her vocabulary, and normalize her voice. I packed my therapy materials and stood at the end of Jeannie's bed. I wanted to ask her if having regained the ability to speak made her feel less alone, but I knew the notion meant nothing to her. Jeannie didn't appreciate the gift of communication at this stage in her recovery, but one day, I hoped, she would. She was smoothing the front of her T-shirt, sucking her stomach inward to a concave shape.

"I'm going now, Jeannie. You know today was our last session, right?"

She didn't look up.

"I hope you get better, maybe get out of here, go to Guernsey one day." I smiled. "Jeannie?"

I extended my hand to shake hers, but she spooked and recoiled. With my outreached hand I waved, turned, and left the room.

Meg and I hugged, and I thanked her for her support. Then, I made my way down the enclosed stairwell. It was an unseasonably cold October day, the sun vanquished by the wind and clouds. I felt a heaviness overcome me. I let my briefcase fall and dropped down on the metal step. The spectacular success and failure of my efforts crashed down on me.

I leaned my head against the cage and looked through the chain-link mesh. The leaves on the trees in the garden below had turned to gold and rust. I thought about my long career in speech therapy and the calling I'd always felt to do my part in alleviating a terrible, essential human loneliness. My patients with communication disorders experienced isolation in its most painful and poignant form. I'd spent over thirty years trying to open channels of communication for them. I'd wanted to do the same for Jeannie.

My mind wandered to something Meg had said in our first conversation. When Jeannie began to eat, after years of being fed through a tube, she began with one raisin. A raisin—it was truly the best unit of measure for gauging her recovery. Progress was agonizingly slow, the changes small and hard won, but they were changes all the same and change meant hope. If I didn't believe that, I would have given up years ago.

I sat on the step for a long while, though I felt cold. Soon, I became aware of noises emanating from the windows of the adolescent ward. There was shouting and moaning and the sound of hands pounding on a door. I pulled myself to standing, gathered my briefcase, and walked away for the last time.

....

Miriam Mandel Levi is a Canadian-trained speech language pathologist who has been living in Israel for the past twenty-two years. "Jeannie" is her first published work.

AN AMERICAN BOY

Candy Schulman

A month after passing his PhD oral exams in neuropsychology, a young man is diagnosed with schizophrenia and admitted to a psychiatric unit. Now he and his family must learn to work together as they navigate the treacherous and unpredictable waters of mental illness.

Will's apartment was a hodgepodge: mismatched cups and glassware; ancient furniture handed down to him by his grandmothers; a sagging upholstered chair; a mattress on the floor; homemade curtains sewn from sheets; old pipes and peeling paint. Even his clothes were frumpy, worn out . . . nothing you'd expect from a single man under forty, who'd once been a brown belt in karate and a reporter for his college newspaper.

My husband and I went through his closets and drawers, uncomfortable with this forced intimacy. "Just close up the apartment," Will had insisted. "I don't want anything. I can't explain it, but I have my reasons."

Yet we took a few things: a photocopy machine, paperbacks whose pages had yellowed. Most importantly, my husband had come to his younger brother's railroad flat in Park Slope, Brooklyn, to retrieve the irreplaceable.

"Maybe he'll want them someday," David said dubiously, packing a suitcase with his brother's birth certificate, a college diploma from the University of Pennsylvania, his PhD dissertation, a passport, even love letters.

There were tears in David's eyes when he lifted up a photograph album. "My brother's high school rock band," he said.

Will and his friends—all of them so vibrant and alive. Today his friends are lawyers and doctors and businessmen; they have children; they take vacations and travel; they play tennis and Scrabble. Today Will rarely leaves his parents' Arizona apartment, where he has been living for the past year.

David closed the small suitcase. "My brother's life," he said, "in one small bag."

Will was diagnosed with schizophrenia fifteen years ago. The label was changed to atypical schizophrenia because he functioned at too high a level to fit into the usual category of disease that produces delusions, hallucinations, and disordered thinking.

His first symptoms went unnoticed; he'd always been offbeat. During the 1960s, he blended in with the counterculture. His attempts at "finding himself" didn't seem eccentric for the time. He earned a BA from an Ivy League college. He was a lifeguard in Key West and wanted to write a novel, like Hemingway. Later, he worked in a molybdenum mine in Colorado, lived in a yurt, and was a San Francisco construction worker before hitchhiking back east.

Then he started talking about Kundalini yoga. He'd always been interested in Eastern philosophies, and having practiced yoga myself, I listened as Will explained: "There's this force in your spine. When it's good, it flows up to your brain and provides enlightenment."

He was following the practices of Bhagwan Shree Rajneesh, who would later plead guilty to immigration violations and be expelled from this country to be remembered mostly for heading an Oregon commune where he acquired possessions from four thousand followers and drove Rolls-Royces.

"I may go to India," Will continued. "I need to correct the force in my spine. I tried to reach enlightenment, but I messed up and now it's completely off course. I tried to look into the third eye."

"I see," I said, although I did not.

Will was finishing his PhD dissertation on aphasia in adults (the inability to articulate ideas or comprehend language because of brain damage). He'd also worked with a leading researcher, splitting the brains of pigeons to investigate how the independent workings of both halves might help victims of stroke and epilepsy. Pretty esoteric stuff, especially to his salesman father and his mother, who'd completed only one year of college. But they were proud of him.

Although Will's quest to correct the spiritual force in his spine continued to distress him, he seemed like any other "normal" young man. He enjoyed political debates, endorsed programs for the disadvantaged, and criticized his father when he talked about minorities as cultural stereotypes. He went to the movies, listened to music, read Nietzsche, Jung, and Hesse. He was an avid baseball fan—albeit for the Yankees when I preferred the Mets, something we kidded each other about. He even went out on dates once in a while.

"I just hope he gets *married*," his mother said, yearning for her son to share her values of a typical middle-class life.

A month after he passed his PhD orals in neuropsychology, Will started refusing to eat or drink. He became extremely agitated. Only after four hours of convincing from a psychiatrist friend did Will finally go to the hospital where he was admitted to a psychiatric unit. Diagnosis: schizophrenia. He paced his hospital room, not knowing where he was. Will was shot full of strong antipsychotic drugs.

Two weeks later, the doctors realized he had a broken neck after his repeated complaints of discomfort. Moved to a medical floor, he was rushed to an operating room where a "halo" was installed: a circular wire apparatus drilled into his forehead to keep his neck straight while it healed. It was a miracle he hadn't become paralyzed. A miracle he'd survived at all. Information leaked out in stages. First the family saw the alarming psychotic symptoms. Next came the neck pain, which we assumed stemmed from a leap he'd suddenly confessed having taken from a moving truck on Third Avenue in Manhattan after hitching a ride to a place we'd never discover. And only after going through his possessions in his apartment a year later, I read his suicide note; he claimed in trying to get the enlightenment force up to his brain, he'd twirled his neck around for a half hour despite the pain.

The family began to search for answers, but research on schizophrenia is complex and evolving. As a trained psychologist, I tried to disseminate information as best I could. According to the National Institute of Mental Health, schizophrenia affects 3.5 million people in the United States, 1 percent of the population. The disease is more common in developed countries. Although no cultural or geographical group is immune, research psychiatrist Dr. E. Fuller Torrey observes the highest incidence of schizophrenia in southern Ireland, Croatia, and some Scandinavian countries. It is unclear why the lowest rates are in Italy, Spain, remote parts of Africa, and Southeast Asia. In a pattern that suggests cultural overtones, Europeans tend toward delusions of poisoning or religious guilt, whereas in Japan delusions are more often related to the fear of slander.

No one cause has yet been discovered, and indeed, schizophrenia may be many illnesses combined. Researchers today theorize it springs from a combination of genetic and environmental factors. Schizophrenia runs in families, and there is a higher incidence of the illness in those conceived during famines and in families from lower socioeconomic groups.

Once thought of as a psychological condition for which mothers were to blame, schizophrenia is now viewed as a brain disorder, a chemical imbalance possibly occurring in fetal development even though symptoms don't emerge until after puberty—perhaps a genetic predisposition triggered by stress. Modern use of MRIs reveals the brains of many schizophrenics to have structural abnormalities.

In 1991, the *New York Times* reported:

> People born immediately after an influenza epidemic may be at significantly higher risk for developing schizophrenia as adults than babies born in years without high flu rates. . . . It is well documented that people born in late winter and early spring are more likely to develop schizophrenia than those born at other times of the year. Since influenza peaks during the winter months, scientists have suggested a viral link.

Will was born in January.

Scientists continue to explore the relationship between flu and schizophrenia. In 2007 Paul Patterson, a neuroscientist at the California Institute of Technology, discussed how flu virus could cause schizophrenia, providing direction for future research. Dr. Alan Brown, of Columbia University, reported that up to 14 percent of schizophrenia cases would not have occurred had influenza in early to mid-pregnancy been avoided, and that viruses and other infections in the first trimester of pregnancy could increase schizophrenia risk as much as 700%.

Here is what we know for sure: schizophrenia interferes with the ability to think clearly, control emotions, and relate to others.

My family is always searching for the answer to the unanswerable question: Why? Why did Will have such potential, only to spend his days now staring into space?

"He has no life," his mother often moans. "*Why?*"

After three weeks in the psychiatric ward, Will was discharged, armed with medications and referrals for outpatient treatment. When we took him to a restaurant for dinner, people stared at the unsightly metal halo surrounding his head and secured onto his chest with long bars. I'm sure there's a story explaining all the details of Will's broken neck and why exactly he stopped eating, but no one knows the truth. Not even us.

Will had been brought up as a Reform Jew in an affluent New Jersey suburb, and in college he was an atheist. During his illness, he began attending a church in the South Bronx where he was sometimes the only white person and always the only Jew. He never told us; we found out because once he refused to leave the church after the service, and the pastor called an ambulance to take him to Metropolitan Hospital where we found him incoherent, dehydrated, in tattered clothing, clutching a Bible.

Psychiatrists made various suggestions: psychotherapy coupled with antipsychotic drugs; antipsychotic drugs alone; long-term inpatient treatment in a private psychiatric hospital; residential treatment at bucolic farms upstate, where Will would, unfortunately, be among a population "much sicker" than he was. What they agreed on: his family had to provide a supportive, nonthreatening environment to aid in his recovery.

Will resisted psychiatric treatment, claiming, "Believe me, I have a *spiritual* problem. If I can only reverse the flow in my spine . . ."

Inexplicably he brought homeless people into his apartment. He gave them keys, money, even his wallet, and then disappeared for days. Did voices instruct him to house the needy? Was it part of his religious delusions? Will's father would call the police to search for his missing son. Once, my husband received a call at work from Montefiore Hospital in the Bronx; although there was no money in Will's wallet, they'd found David's number, and would he come right away?

On another occasion, before we were wise enough to obtain a set of keys to Will's apartment, his father had to go there when Will wouldn't answer his phone. (We later found out he'd ripped the phone right out of the wall.) Entering a neighbor's apartment, his father climbed onto the fire escape and through Will's window, where he found his son, a zombie wearing a brown wig, sitting cross-legged on his bed. He had to change the locks to make sure people Will had given his keys to wouldn't return. A limping vagrant showed up at the door saying, "But I just got out of the hospital, man. Will promised I could stay here . . ."

His father called Will's boss, saying he had the flu. Due to the stigma of mental illness, many people hide their condition from employers for risk of losing their jobs. Sometimes Will was fired after repeated bouts of "flu," but he always managed to recover and get a new job, such as performing psychological evaluations and implementing behavior-modification techniques for developmentally disabled adults at a clinic in Washington Heights, a low-paying, unglamorous position that many PhDs wouldn't bother with.

Each hospitalization stabilized him with drugs that control symptoms but do not provide a cure. Once Will was discharged, he'd again refuse to take his medication—not only because of the side effects, but because the delusions were convincing Will he could find solace elsewhere. In New York State, patients' civil rights are protected by the Mental Hygiene Law. We couldn't commit Will because he wasn't posing "a substantial threat of harm" to himself or others. More than once David or his father stood over him in one hospital or another, practically yelling that he admit himself by signing a Voluntary Evaluation/ Admission form.

"My son needs help," his father would say in frustration. "Why can't someone *force* him into the hospital?"

His mother would say, "I just want him to have some kind of *life*."

"I hope he doesn't get fired again," his father would say.

"Yes," his mother would agree. "What'll happen if he loses his health insurance?"

Most managed care plans won't pay for long-term care, and once we got him in, Will was released as soon as he was medically stable, always shrewdly promising the doctors and us that he'd take his medication. He did not.

"The drugs make me sleepy," Will complained. "They distort my thinking. There are side effects."

Twitching, muscle spasms, impotence, and tardive dyskinesia— involuntary movements particularly of the lower face. Although antipsychotic drugs are a panacea for some, reducing or eliminating symptoms, many patients resist tolerating the range of side effects, from dry mouth to dizziness.

"Why won't he take his medicine?" his mother would wail.

"It's part of his illness," David would say again and again, the same conversation repeated day after day, year after year. Will kept insisting that he wasn't physically ill and that, therefore, Western medicine couldn't help him. Although it has been painful for us to adjust to this new Will and lower our expectations of him—to realize that just *showering* is almost as huge an accomplishment as finishing his dissertation—perhaps no one feels it as deeply as his mother. Mothers had long been blamed for causing schizophrenia, and it's difficult to escape the self-imposed guilt that results from old stereotypes.

He had delusions that he could cure himself. And so he went to church. Stopped eating meat. Stopped seeing women. He even stopped seeing movies. And he started writing a book.

"One day I'll let you read it," he said. "One day you'll understand."

When we cleaned out his apartment, we found the book, and tried to read some sections. It was written in a florid prose. None of it made any sense, but it was voluminous: one thousand pages. The first line: "I will save the world." He was convinced that enlightenment would free him from the voices and the terrifying symptoms none of us could ever fully understand.

A year after Will's first inpatient stay, the police called to tell us they had picked him up in the South Bronx and taken him to Lincoln Hospital. He had been sitting in a trancelike state on a park bench for twenty-four hours when someone notified them. We arranged for an ambulance to drive him to St. Vincent's where his doctor was affiliated.

Despite the frosty March temperature, he was wearing a thin denim jacket and no gloves. "How do you feel?" we asked him.

His mouth moved, but no words emerged. His lips were cracked and chapped. Four days' growth of beard surrounded his face, and his reddened fingers held a paperback Bible.

"Will. Are you okay?"

He shut his eyes.

He was led toward the emergency room entrance, but the ambulance driver caught up to his father and said, "Next of kin? Payment is a hundred and fifty bucks."

"He has insurance," his father said.

"We don't take insurance. Cash or check."

Inside, Will sat in a wheelchair. A woman whose husband had been stabbed was alternating screams with rapid-fire Spanish. A resident was trying to convince her to give him the knife she was holding. Her blouse was streaked with blood.

Will's mouth moved, but no sound yet.

"You'll feel better when the medication takes effect," his mother said above the screams. "See what happens when you don't take your pills? When's the last time you had a shower?"

Will smiled. His hair was oily, stringy. He held his Bible tighter. He looked like the man who'd sat next to me on the subway the week before: a disheveled, mumbling soul in torn clothing who caused passengers to move away in fear. How many times had Will entered subway cars like a madman?

"Oh Will," his mother said. "What's to become of you?"

A teardrop fell out of the corner of his left eye.

"Have you paid your rent?" his father asked.

Suddenly Will opened his eyes. "I'm a born-again Christian now," he said with an unsure grin.

Last time it was a Seventh-day Adventist.

"Go read your Bible," he continued. "There's still time. I went to the Bronx to preach."

"Don't you think you took a risk spending the night in that neighborhood?" his mother asked.

"The Messiah is coming."

"To the *South Bronx*?" she asked incredulously.

"The Messiah is coming," he repeated.

"I hope he comes soon," his father said, "for your benefit."

Hospitalization number nine. Paranoid, delusional, had not eaten in days. A patient with a long history who'd be out on the streets soon and, before long, back again.

"He doesn't have many hospital days left on his insurance," his mother worried.

"Good thing it's December," said his father. "The new year will bring ninety more hospital days."

Will wasn't in terrible shape this time. We'd seen him ripping the IV out of his arm, screaming at nurses, urinating on the floor, spitting at doctors. We'd seen him in straitjackets, and we'd seen him cry like an infant. Eventually the drugs would chase the bad voices away. Tomorrow he'd be walking around. Nurses would make him shower and shave. He'd apologize for all the trouble he'd caused. We'd play checkers or gin rummy. He'd stop talking about religion.

Until next time.

The family shuffled Will from psychiatrist to psychiatrist. He almost died from an allergic reaction to Haldol, a drug given to him upon admission one Christmas at Columbia University Medical Center. A wonderful resident there told us he wasn't schizophrenic, but had "periodic catatonia," not widely known in the United States. Periodic catatonia frequently presented itself with religious delusions and periods of not talking; often, patients recovered quickly from episodes and went back to work. The disorder had a better prognosis than schizophrenia, and patients often responded positively to lithium.

His mother was always clinging to any new hope—*Maybe this was the cure!*

"Don't have high hopes," the doctor warned us. "Will doesn't accept the diagnosis."

And from his hospital bed in a prison-cell-sized room near Harlem, Will railed, "I refuse! Lithium can kill a person."

I tried to reason with him to no avail.

We were given the name of an expert in periodic catatonia, but Will would not agree to a consultation. He continually denied his illness. And we'll never know what the voices inside his head were instructing him to do—and not to do.

"He's stubborn," his mother complained. "Like his father."

"He's sick," we had to remind her and ourselves.

His parents took him to a rabbi. Once they even considered seeing a psychic known to specialize in such cases. We looked for patterns: he seemed to get "sick" between Christmas and his birthday and, in summer, around the time of our wedding anniversary. When he was supposed to be an usher at a cousin's wedding, he went into the hospital instead; was it too upsetting to watch his cousin begin a happy life? Friends and relatives—all concerned at first and providing bedside vigils—eventually lost interest, or patience, or courage. Repeatedly he decompensated. He learned to show up on his parents' doorstep and meekly say, "I don't feel well. Can I stay here for a while?"

Once he showed up with a copy of the Old Testament. "At least it's the right religion," his mother said with a sigh. "What's going to happen when I'm not here anymore?"

During moments of despair, David will turn to me and confess his own worries: Will he have the strength to care for Will after his parents die? The moral and financial responsibilities are daunting. He can understand why there are so many people on the streets; he understands what would drive entire families to give up.

Saturday, 3:00 a.m., the telephone rang. "I'm feeling ill," Will's voice said. "Could I come over?"

His parents had just retired to Arizona, and Will had encouraged them to do so even though for the past five years they'd prevented many hospitalizations by finally convincing him to come to their home when he first felt the symptoms.

Fifteen minutes later he called to say he was okay, he wouldn't be coming over. At 5:00 a.m. he rang our doorbell.

David gave him Mellaril, making sure that he was drinking water lest he dehydrate. Because it has been associated with arrhythmias and even sudden death, Mellaril tends to be prescribed to schizophrenics who don't respond to other drugs.

Will slept on our living room couch until breakfast, which he refused to eat. "I want to go home now," he said.

That night there was a message on our answering machine from him: "Thank you for having me. I apologize for disturbing you."

The next calls came from Arizona; his parents had called Will and left messages, which remained unreturned. David ran to Will's apartment to find him in a semi-catatonic state. He roused him from sleep, made him take more Mellaril, and forced him to drink water, threatening him with hospitalization if he didn't agree.

I received the next call. "I'm on my way to the airport," Will said calmly. "I don't feel well. I have to go to Arizona."

"Are you okay?" I asked lamely. "I mean, can I come with you to the airport, at least? I'll ride in the cab with you."

"No, I'm fine," Will said. "But thanks. Thanks for everything."

He'd become dependent on his parents' care, their doling out medication as if he were a little kid. At the age of thirty-nine, he moved in with his parents. He felt safer with them than on his own. He needed to be taken care of, and unlike the parents of so many other schizophrenics, his were willing to accept this lifelong challenge and burden.

During a visit to Arizona the next Christmas, we watched old family movies. Will and David, riding bikes outside their suburban ranch house. Romping in the snow, tossing a football, eating ice cream, play-fighting. Two all-American boys.

Afterward we talked and joked, while Will kept getting up and going into his room. Five minutes later he'd come back, walk around the dining room table, touch a chair, move the chair, and then sit in it. Then he'd repeat it again. We wanted to take him out for lunch, but he was washing and drying his clothes. We waited an hour until he was done.

"His doctor says he feels he's dirty, that he's caused impure thoughts in his head," explained his mother. "He washes his clothes three times a day. I can't afford the electric bills." She was teary-eyed. "All those years he thought he could 'fix' his problem, and now . . . How can he give up? How can I?"

We took Will to the mall, his major outing for the week. In a store where we were buying holiday presents, the salesclerk cheerfully said, "You two must be brothers. Now let me guess. . . ." She focused on Will. "You're the older one, right?"

He was nearly five years younger than David, but his poor muscle tone, bulging stomach, and sallow skin tone gave a clue to the more complex story.

He no longer gets that "wild look" in his eyes, keying us in to an impending psychotic episode. Sometimes he behaves like a little kid. Two weeks after my birthday, he sent me a card saying, "I'm sorry I missed your birthday. I want to buy you a present." I nearly cried, thinking of the thoughtful gifts he used to give me when he was still interested in reading classics by Hemingway and listening to rock music from the sixties.

Recently, on the way home from yet another doctor's visit with his parents, he began to sob in the back seat.

"I'm sorry," he told them. "Forgive me."

"We love you," his mother said.

"I'm sorry . . . and thank you. For everything you've done."

Will's mother knew he was always most sweet when he was most ill and most irascible during independent periods of "recovery." She turned to him and asked, "What are you going to do with the rest of your life?"

"I don't know," he said. "I'm disabled."

"What's going to happen to you after I'm gone?"

"I don't know."

. . .

No one—neither the family nor doctors—can predict the course of Will's illness. We're all pioneering an unknown landscape, an arduous hike with a terrain full of unexpected twists, surprises, and setbacks.

David looks after his brother's financial affairs while Will is living with his parents. He feels guilty when he becomes angry with Will—because he's sick, because he can't reason, because he saps so much energy from the family.

Sometimes, when Will has taken a nap on our bed, I've hesitated to use the same pillow, as if I might catch something. This is irrational, but I vacillate between empathy and disgust. Even for a mental health professional, it's difficult to shake off old notions about illnesses.

I think of him whenever I listen to Mozart's *The Magic Flute*, a CD Will gave me for no reason at all, back when he enjoyed sharing the music he loved. Unlike Pamina in the opera, Will has not really been kidnapped. But will we ever find a magic flute to guide us to the place where the real Will is being held?

Three years after moving to Arizona, Will begins to improve, almost miraculously. No one can explain his sudden plunge into mental illness, and no one could have predicted his entry back into the world. It happens soon after his father has died from cancer, the type of stress that would cause most schizophrenics to decompensate. Instead, he suddenly announces that he will get a job. But first he returns to Brooklyn, on a quest to retrieve his belongings from his long-ago abandoned apartment, which he believes are all still in the same spot. He will need them, he says, for the new apartment he plans to rent all by himself.

"Will," I suggest gently, trying not to convey how ridiculous he sounds, "your landlord must have given—or thrown—everything away."

"He probably called the Salvation Army to come pick everything up," David adds.

Will shakes his head. "I know you can't understand this, but I left everything there for a reason. And I know it's all waiting for me."

He even has his key. I try to persuade him that someone has undoubtedly changed the locks until I remind myself that it makes no sense to argue with Will. It's easy to forget, to try to reason with him.

He goes uptown to his former apartment and returns, empty-handed. When I ask what happened, he only says, "My landlord put my things in storage somewhere. He's holding them for me until the time is right."

I try to hide my dubious reaction.

"It's part of the plan," Will says.

Back in Arizona, he writes his résumé and begins answering "help wanted" ads. He is hired at a nonprofit that mentors at-risk teenagers. We don't know how he explained his unemployed years, how he interviewed so convincingly, or how he will react to the demands of a full-time job. He joins a gym, buys attractive new clothes and a zippy sports car. Every morning he showers, eats breakfast, and drives to work. Like everyone else.

After more than a decade of monk-like celibacy, Will begins dating several women. When he doesn't come home one night, Will's mother worries that he is psychotic somewhere and in danger. Turns out he was spending the night at a woman's apartment.

He is angry that his mother questions him so closely, like a sixteen-year-old who's just gotten his license and is staying out beyond curfew. Will talks again about getting his own apartment. Not immediately . . . but soon.

Today, if you met him at a party, he would engage in a conversation about sports or politics. He'd stay clear of anything threatening, such as his illness or emotions. You probably wouldn't know anything was wrong. But his mother notices a bottle of anti-psychotic drugs in the medicine cabinet, slowly dwindling and being refilled. Will medicates himself just enough to quell the disturbing voices, even though doctors tell him it's better if the drugs are taken consistently, on a regular basis. And periodically he's off to Las Vegas, believing he has finally devised a system for blackjack, or roulette, or craps. Once he wins $10,000 on a Super Bowl bet, and we try to encourage him to save it, buy stock, put it in an IRA. The next time he loses it all and more.

"You need to save for your retirement," we tell him.

He laughs. "Don't worry. I'll be taken care of."

By whom? A girlfriend? A spiritual force? Public assistance? He fluctuates from making sense to revealing the underpinnings of a mind that's foreign to us, neurological differences that make him sound sane and controlled in one moment, odd and irrational the next.

He makes another trip to New Jersey for a high school reunion, and we have lunch together. Instead of carrying a Bible, he holds a copy of Proust's *Swann's Way*. He chats about his job, how he works with teenagers who are troubled. I listen to him and express praise that he is working and doing so well. I am astounded that he has made such progress, against all odds. Atypical schizophrenia, by all means. What's in a label, anyway? Aren't we all atypical in our own ways?

After I leave to return to work, I sneak one last look at him back in the café. I wonder if he thinks about or even remembers his previous life before the chemical imbalance overcame him. Once he was an all-American suburban boy: smart, athletic, laughing with friends, squabbling with his brother, planning for the future.

Parents can never predict which path their children will take, yet they try their best to guide children into the American fabric of aspiration and dreams: get a good education, work hard, find a soul mate, buy a house, have kids. Parents can control and influence, passing on their values—to a point. Sometimes luck and genetics prevail over love and comfort.

Not everyone is destined to fit into the successful model valued by our society. Sometimes atypical personalities are revered, like Steve Jobs. Will, like so many others, hid his disturbing symptoms from his family during college and grad school. Then he spent decades struggling through a devastating illness. Now he looks calm, even "normal," reading a paperback book and sipping his coffee, perhaps spending a few moments contemplating life.

Is this a happy ending? Yes and no. Will's family remains guarded. Although we are thrilled that Will is doing "so well," we never use the words "recovered" or "cured." We know better than that: the next episode might be months away, or weeks, or even days. Tomorrow that dreaded phone call might come, but in the meantime, we welcome the respite. And hope that Will does, too.

....

Candy Schulman's essays, articles, and humor have appeared in publications and anthologies including the New York Times, *the* Washington Post, McSweeney's, Salon.com, Parents, Brain Child, *and* The Forward. *She received a Best Essay Award from the American Society of Journalists and Authors for her* Chicago Tribune *essay on caring for elderly parents, an excerpt from her memoir. She has an MA in psychology and is a writing professor at The New School.*

I'M NOT A NOUN EITHER

Tom Mallouk

When does a diagnosis become a label? A psychotherapist tries unconventional paths—including Tae kwon do—to find common ground with a schizophrenic patient who insists, "I am not a schizophrenic."

I was fired from my first two jobs in psychology after twice making the fatal error of talking to people.

In the first case, I was a college student working as a research assistant in a sleep lab. My job entailed placing electrodes on subjects and hooking them up to various machines that would measure eye movements, respirations, and muscle tone while they slept. During different stages of sleep, I was to wake them up and record their dreams.

Psychology is, as are all social sciences, a "soft" science. Natural sciences, such as physics and chemistry, are considered "hard" sciences. Researchers working in the hard sciences take great pains to control environments, ensuring that nothing influences the results of an experiment as they isolate phenomena and support or disprove hypotheses. In an attempt to gain legitimacy, the social sciences have borrowed wholesale the values of the natural sciences. But humans turn out to be unlike rocks and germs in fundamental ways. Since humans are experimenting with other humans, the effort to keep undue influence out of psychological research has been, to say the least, daunting.

Shortly after I began work at the sleep lab, the study's director appeared while I was preparing the machines and chatting with the subject during this often tedious process. The next day the director called an emergency staff meeting. He was horrified that I had been talking to a subject while preparing him for the study. The director must have assumed I knew the proper protocol, but I was a senior in college and had taken just one psychology course. My understanding of the controlled environment was, at that time, very limited. I didn't know we weren't supposed to talk to the subjects.

After the meeting, I was summoned to the office of one of the senior people and fired.

I was, of course, devastated. Fortunately, the person assigned the thankless task of giving me the ax was kind. He informed me there were many other areas of psychology that might better suit me. Since I liked talking to people, he said, clinical psychology might be a nice fit.

Indeed the art of dialogue is the psychotherapist's principal skill. My first job in the clinical arena should have been right up my alley, but instead it was even worse than my initial exposure to the field in sleep research.

Shortly after graduation, I got a job as a counselor for the chronically mentally ill. State hospitals were closing and patients were being placed in intensive outpatient programs. Residents lived in apartments while attending clinics during the day. This type of arrangement was part of an ongoing progression in the mental hygiene field to avoid warehousing the mentally ill in large state institutions, where they often became permanently isolated from the community.

As in many of these efforts, the impulse was noble, but the execution was faulty. In this particular program, the psychiatrist who hired me was clearly afraid of the patients. I never saw him directly interact with any of the patients, and he seemed furtive and anxious whenever he passed through the patient areas on his way to his third-floor office. His fear was unfounded. These patients were not dangerous. Their lives were mostly sad and empty. Many had been lobotomized and all were heavily medicated.

Each morning one of the counselors began the day by convening everyone in a large meeting room to outline the activities for the day and address any issues that might have arisen in the previous twenty-four hours.

When I arrived for work one day, I was informed that one of the patients had committed suicide the night before. The patients needed to be informed, and it was my turn to convene the daily meeting.

I started by telling them that something sad had happened. I told them of the suicide and went on to say, "All of us have experienced the kind of darkness that 'Jane' must have known, but suicide is not a solution."

I told the patients the truth. I *did* know Jane's darkness. I had experienced a devastating drug-induced psychosis a few years earlier, and as part of my recovery, I had gone through an unremitting suicidal depression. My friends had helped protect me from my suicidal wishes, and I hoped to create a similar sort of support group for the patients by showing them we all—patients and staff alike—shared in similar struggles.

That afternoon I was fired. The psychiatrist was clearly shaken, and who could blame him? There was, after all, a dead patient. But he wasn't focused on the patient we'd lost. He was more concerned with my comments in the community meeting. He believed I had breached the boundary between staff and patients, and such close relationships, he said, could only increase the anxiety of the residents. He believed the staff should appear as somehow invulnerable. To state or even intimate we knew of any "darkness" made depression and suicidal thoughts more acceptable. The suicide, to the psychiatrist's mind, needed to be banished.

My inclination to communicate and identify with patients came naturally. I grew up in a family steeped in mental illness. My father was given to fits of violence, especially toward me, and my mother was hospitalized several times, receiving insulin shock therapy in the 1950s and electroconvulsive therapy in the 1960s. She had what was then called manic depression but is now referred to as bipolar disorder. She drank heavily to manage her moods and eventually developed alcoholism, which contributed to her premature death at the age of fifty-one.

In spite of these obstacles, my parents produced six children, all of whom are better adjusted psychologically and emotionally. And even though I suffered a terrible psychosis, I recovered with the help of friends, family, and adequate treatment to become in my post-psychosis life a person with greater capacity to enjoy life.

I knew experientially but did not yet understand theoretically that what we call mental illness is isolating and stigmatizing. My family certainly understood we were different from our neighbors, who were not shaking the walls of their homes with emotional outbursts. I felt sheepish when I left the house and imagined what people thought of me and us, but my siblings and I had each other and a large extended family that mitigated the sense of isolation.

My childhood instilled in me a powerful need to understand people and a strong inclination to connect to them, especially those who are struggling. The day program patients were not that different from my parents and were certainly no different from those I had met during my hospitalization. Despite what the director said, I knew that forming a community could effectively attenuate the threat of suicide, which is the ultimate isolation and attack on the self. Even though I'd once again lost my job, I'd think back to that meeting as a defining moment in my career as a psychotherapist. "We are in this together," I expressed to the patients. "And we are not bad for experiencing profound darkness."

Three years after my second firing I was visiting my future wife during her surgical rotation in medical school when I overheard two surgeons discussing their day. One was telling the other he had done "two gallbladders" while the other countered that he had done "three hernias."

This struck me as an interesting way to talk. These organs had seemingly not been attached to human beings. The medical students had all just witnessed their first surgeries, and a conversation ensued about the surgical theater and how the area to be operated on was visually isolated from the rest of the patient's body. There are some antiseptic reasons for such separation, but the students agreed that covering the rest of the patient's body was useful in blocking out the momentousness of cutting into another human being. The surgeons' references to "gallbladders" and "hernias" could be seen as an extension of the need to depersonalize the process, to isolate the offending organ from the human organism.

In the medical field, symptoms are evidence of some disease process. The practice of medicine involves diagnosing the disease and, ideally, curing it. The symptom, in other words, is evidence of the disease and its elimination is part of the cure.

In the intensive outpatient program, the psychiatrist—operating from the medical model—wanted to eliminate any evidence of the disease that caused the suicide, including me and my intimation that a staff member had experienced the kind of darkness that led to the suicide. By eliminating the suicide altogether and firing me, the psychiatrist hoped to "cure" the program of its sickness. But what if psychological symptoms are very different from physical ones? What if psychological symptoms contain important information about the process of the cure? Would it then be possible that the elimination of the symptom would undermine the likelihood of a cure? Hiding the suicide would then interfere with the healing process for the other patients.

My experience in the day program and subsequent years of work and research have revealed that embedded in the way professionals think about mental illness are isolating and demeaning tendencies that inadvertently exacerbate the very problems the field is trying to correct. No psychotherapist worth the title would ever chat with a colleague about having seen two depressives, three bipolars, and one schizoaffective before lunch. Yet today in the mail, I received a brochure touting a continuing education program called "Assessing, Managing and Treating Personality Disorders: A Gathering of Experts." Clearly, the language used in this brochure dehumanizes those who have these disorders by reducing them to nothing beyond their own suffering. We are not treating the people, the diction implies. We're treating the illnesses.

Even when the process of diagnosis is at its best, the mental health professional may still claim expertise in the relational environment that is supposed to cultivate healing. The clinician is placed in a one-up position where power rather than connection becomes the underlying dynamic. Most psychic suffering has its roots in early development through misattunement between infant (underdeveloped nervous system) and caregiver (presumably more developed nervous system). When the clinician adopts a posture of superior knowledge and remains disengaged from the patient in order to promote or maintain "professional objectivity," the context of the therapeutic encounter runs the risk of reenacting the relational ruptures that created the problem in the first place.

What I knew from my own recovery was that medication helped manage my acute symptoms and seeing my psychiatrist gave me hope that I would not always feel as bad as I felt in the aftermath of the psychosis. But what literally saved my life was a community of friends who were aware that I was struggling and made it a point of keeping me engaged. If a meal was being prepared in the apartment below mine, I was encouraged to bring a bottle of soda and come for dinner. If a group was going to a concert or a movie, someone would prod me to join the crowd. I was a wounded whale and my friends were a coordinated pod nudging me toward the surface whenever I started to sink.

During my final year of doctoral training, I was working in Philadelphia as an intern in a psychotherapy clinic connected to a school for learning-disabled kids. My office was only a few blocks from our home, so every Thursday I spent a hurried lunch hour food shopping for my little family. My wife, who was in her final year of residency, was pregnant with our first child, and it seemed like we already had three mouths to feed.

. On a particularly cold day, I raced through the aisles and got myself on a short checkout line when a woman who seemed about my age got in line behind me. She wore a lightweight wool coat and had one of those two-wheeled carts people use to walk home with their groceries. It was perhaps five degrees outside, and I began to wonder how far she had to go.

I felt awkward because I didn't want her to get the wrong impression, and I knew any side trip would cause me to be late getting back to work. Still, the thought of anyone having to walk too far in that cold was disconcerting. So I struck up a conversation. Before long she told me that her car had stalled, but that she "only" had eight blocks to walk. I offered her a ride, which she gratefully accepted.

Eventually, I told her I was a psychologist, and her eyes lit up. She wanted to know where I worked and what kind of people I saw. There was real urgency in her questions and, as we drove toward her home, she asked if I would be willing to talk to her brother-in-law.

Steve was living with her and her husband and was very disturbed but would not talk to a professional because of "what happened in New York." As we were driving the last half block, I told her that if she could get Steve to me, I would be happy to talk with him. I pulled into their driveway and was astonished by the sight of a young man dressed in shorts and a tee shirt attempting to wash the windows of her stalled car.

Not only was Steve fearfully underdressed for the weather, but he was also dribbling massive amounts of mucus into his mustache, which was frozen in place. As we unloaded the groceries, Steve and I were introduced and arrangements were made for us to have a conversation the next day.

This young man fit the classic description for schizophrenia with blunted affect, inattention to basic grooming, bizarre facial expression, and inappropriate social behavior. He had, in fact, been hospitalized at one of the most respected psychiatric hospitals in New York. Against medical advice, he had signed himself out of the program because he objected to his diagnosis and had stopped taking his medication. Within days he was acutely psychotic but unwilling to speak with professionals.

I sensed our meeting outside of an institutional setting as well as my inferior status as an intern rather than a doctor contributed to Steve's willingness to speak with me.

He opened our first session with the announcement, "I am not a schizophrenic!"

"Fair enough," I replied. "I am not a noun either." And so we began.

In our sessions, Steve mirrored the reports I received from his family. He exhibited periods of lucidity punctuated by episodes of bizarre behavior. At times, there was some connection to a shared social reality as in the case of cleaning the windshield, but often there was no apparent link to the world beyond his psychotic truth. The one constant was his off-putting demeanor. His speech was always pressured, his hair disheveled, and his eyes bugged out of his head.

Usually what someone says at the beginning of the first encounter is crucial to the future therapeutic course. What I learned from Steve was that as long as we did not refer to him as a "schizophrenic," we could talk about nearly anything.

Over time, I noticed some rhyme and reason to his bizarre outbreaks. Once, when the subject of girls came up, he abruptly sat forward in his chair and began what appeared to be the backstroke while looking at the ceiling and humming. Often when we were having a good conversation and I felt a certain warmth developing between us, Steve would interrupt with a word salad or strange facial contortions. Attempts on my part to find out what he was experiencing were unsuccessful.

Typically, Steve's comments would include something abnormal, but rather than confront the anomalies, I would respond to what did make sense. When Steve introduced himself by saying "I am not a schizophrenic," I didn't confront the odd statement by saying, "Are you concerned about being called a schizophrenic?" Instead, I attempted to join him by saying, "I am not a noun either." I wanted to relate rather than confront.

At the time, I couldn't explain my reasoning in theoretical terms. I was working more on instinct than anything, but I've come to believe the process of helping someone with a disorganized and fragmented sense of self move toward greater coherence and integration requires a sense of connection or attunement from the more organized/integrated person to the disorganized/fragmented one. To confront would add to the distress whereas to relate might open a pathway for Steve to become more organized through connection to my more organized self.

My response was similar to the way in which I'd communicated with the group following the suicide at the intensive outpatient program, and I am sure I was taking my cue from my friends who had refused to abandon me. Additionally, by suggesting that schizophrenia was just a noun, I attempted to neutralize the de-meaning quality of the diagnosis.

Steve and I were connecting in a positive way one day when suddenly, something like panic flickered across his face. The next thing I knew he had jumped out of his chair and begun a series of bizarre movements in the middle of my office. He was balancing himself on one foot with his arms extended, looking like the human incarnation of a stork.

"What's that?" I asked him.

"Tae kwon do!" Steve said.

I got up and asked Steve to show me. I imitated his movements while asking him to let me know how well I was doing. The remainder of our session consisted of my first tae kwon do lesson.

At the time, I had no clear idea what guided my behavior. I only knew I couldn't do a lot of things my previous training suggested. I couldn't, for example, make the observation that

Steve had abruptly changed the subject or inquire as to what was going on inside him when he jumped from his chair. I couldn't interpret that the closeness developing between us might have encouraged Steve's interruption and unusual behavior. I certainly couldn't engage in "active listening" since I was not dealing with spoken communication.

Steve couldn't tolerate such an approach, which would only drive him further into his isolation and shame. He needed me to help him create a relational environment that would counteract his tendency to behave in ways that would lead to alienation. That environment needed to invite a sense of connection and be biased in the direction of esteeming him, me, and our efforts. By joining him in the practice of tae kwon do and asking him to instruct me, I was implicitly trying to stay connected to him and honoring him as someone with superior knowledge

For the most part, Steve was incapable of articulating his own experience. He was a follower of Baba Ram Dass, the former Harvard psychology professor turned spiritual teacher, and we talked often about Eastern religions. Steve had been told by Ram Dass himself that the pathway to Atman is through Brahman. I was, of course, skeptical that he was actually in touch with Ram Dass, but later I saw the letters. To say that the pathway to Atman is through Brahman is to suggest that the way to enlightenment is through mundane, everyday activities.

This turned out to be the perfect approach to building a bridge between Steve's tortured experience and his ability to participate in what most of us commonly refer to as reality. During this entire period Steve was unwilling to take medication, and although he had stabilized to some extent, he was unable to find a job or sustain any ongoing social relations with people other than his family.

Using the "pathway to Atman is through Brahman" instruction, we addressed issues like personal hygiene, dressing appropriately, and eating properly. These all fit nicely into the traditions of Buddhism and I had familiarized myself with some of the classic Buddhist parables to help us with the work.

In one such story, the acolyte approaches the master after a long journey and says breathlessly, "Master, I have come to attain enlightenment." The master replies, "Have you eaten?" The devotee answers, "No." The master instructs him to "go and eat a bowl of rice." Somewhat frustrated, the student leaves and returns shortly, a little more calm, and says, "Master, I have come to attain enlightenment." Again the master asks, "Have you eaten?" The student replies, "Yes." The master asks, "Have you cleaned your bowl?" The student answers, "No." "Then go clean your bowl," the master says. The student, obviously irritated, blurts out, "I came a long way and traveled through the night. What does eating rice and cleaning my bowl have to do with attaining enlightenment?" When the student looks to the master for a response, he sees the master has fallen asleep and peevishly goes off to clean his bowl.

So in this way, Steve and I talked about enlightenment as something that could be attained only in submission to the day-to-day requirements of living. And he wasn't the only one who needed these lessons. My wife and I were newly married, and soon we would be parents. I, too, was getting a crash course in the requirements of living.

Before long, we were able to discuss Steve's brain in the same way we could talk about his hair. Both required basic hygiene. Steve's unwashed hair would become greasy and matted, and his bangs would fall over his forehead. This could contribute to acne, which made it difficult to attract girls. Of course, the way you begin to smell when you haven't bathed doesn't help either. So the idea was that your hair has requirements that you need to attend to if you want to attract a girl.

Likewise, your brain has certain basic requirements which you need to attend to in order to help it function in the optimal way.

I explained that Steve was born with a unique sort of brain that gave him the capacity to experience things most people could not, but his brain was also fragile. Understanding the world in more conventional ways was sometimes difficult. Steve had less room for error in his life. He could fight the demands of his special sort of brain, or he could submit to its requirements by taking actions that would allow him to function. In addition to enough sleep, proper diet, and respect for his brain's unique sensitivity to stimuli, I suggested, injections every other week of Prolixin D, an antipsychotic medication, would enable Steve to more readily pursue "right practice."

Once Steve agreed to the medication, things progressed more rapidly. The bimonthly injections increased the likelihood of his compliance and made it unnecessary for him to deal with potential indignity on a daily basis. But as far as I know, he never experienced the medicine in this way because it was embedded in a more benign way of thinking about himself and his unique requirements for living.

From the medical model's perspective, the apparent success of Steve's treatment is a simple matter of persuading him to take medicine to correct the chemical imbalance in his brain. I have no problem with that description as far as it goes, but it is a description bereft of any unique or nuanced meaning in the patient's life.

For people like Steve, it's obvious that taking the proper medicine helps enormously in controlling their symptoms. But the question is what way of thinking about these things maximizes the likelihood that taking medicine will be seen as an act of self-love and esteem and not as something demeaning and isolating?

Most physicians will tell you the biggest problem in getting the therapeutic benefit from medicines is what the medical world calls "compliance." Consider young men who are diagnosed with type 1 diabetes. Adolescents are developmentally disinclined to accept their helplessness or inability to master and control. They are notoriously noncompliant when it comes to taking medication. For males with type 1 diabetes, the morbidity and mortality of their condition is mediated by their willingness to comply with an established medical regimen proven to dramatically extend life and improve its quality. A young man with a diagnosis feels stigmatized and isolated, and his noncompliance is a misguided though noble effort to defend his dignity. These same dynamics are at work in many situations in which the afflicted do not follow established medical recommendations, especially in the case of mental illness.

People generally approach psychotherapy having been injured in a way that leads them to feel isolated and demeaned. For Steve and a number of other individuals, the diagnosis of schizophrenia was itself a psychologically damaging event that exacerbated the isolating and stigmatizing aspects of the illness. The alienation and shame is rarely as obvious as in Steve's situation, but isolation tends to drive a person to behave in many complex ways that have often been described as "manipulative" or "neurotic," terms that also carry demeaning implications. The relevant question when people are distressed should not be "What's wrong with you?" but "What has happened to you?"

The task of psychotherapy should be to dignify the struggle of the client. True connection is one of the many tasks of love, and the relationship between a distressed individual and a mental health professional is no exception. I can say now I'm proud I was fired from my first two mental health positions if it meant for a moment, I was able to relate to another's suffering and become part of a supportive community. We share with those we call mentally ill a common fate and template of repair. Trauma leads all of us to bring an isolating and stigmatizing bias to our experience and self-representations, a bias that is often exacerbated by bias in the culture at large and the conventions of psychotherapeutic practice. Psychotherapy and love must bring a countervailing bias, one that tends toward ennobling the efforts of the injured and fosters relationship in the face of isolation.

....

Tom Mallouk is a writer and psychotherapist, who has been in private practice for more than forty years. He was a Russell Conway Fellow while pursuing his doctorate at Temple University. His poetry chapbook, Nantucket Revisited, *was published by Antrim House in 2013. His poetry and creative nonfiction have appeared in* US1 Worksheets, *the* Schuylkill Valley Journal, Pamphlet, Solstice, *and the* Miami Herald, *among others. In 2010, 2012, and 2013 he was runner-up for Bucks County Poet Laureate. He lives in Doylestown, Pennsylvania, with his wife, Dr. Eileen Engle.*

INDISTINGUISHABLE CHAIRS

Cassie Eaton

After visiting a series of therapists with varying degrees of success, one woman decides to take the healing process into her own hands—with the goal of "surviving, then prevailing, and sometimes triumphing."

The word *recovery* suggests an end to something that ails you. The Substance Abuse and Mental Health Services Association defines it as a process of improving your health and wellness, living a self-directed life, and striving to reach your full potential. But that's just life, isn't it? It's what we are all working for, ill or not.

What does it mean to recover from a mental illness? Should I attempt to reach my full potential *despite* my illness—living like everyone else, shunning this disease that always will be in me? Or should I reach my full potential side by side with my illness—allowing it to propel me into a life I never would have expected? I don't want to *recover*, I want to grow, evolve, and transform through the traumatic experiences brought about by my illness. It's not *recovery* I am aiming for; it's surviving, then prevailing, and sometimes triumphing.

For me, it was my inability to cope with trauma that led to internal growth and post-traumatic evolution. At eighteen, I was diagnosed with borderline personality disorder and bipolar disorder, and now, at thirty years old, I have been given the additional gift of post-traumatic stress disorder. Due to these diagnoses, listed not in order of diagnostic axis but in order of symptom acuity, I have struggled to relate to, participate in, and even be accepted for therapy on many occasions.

I never stuck with therapy long enough for it to work. Or quite possibly I never had the right therapist. I eventually decided that if working with a therapist wasn't going to help me, I should learn as much about therapy as I could on my own, in order to help myself. Rather than a therapeutic process of recovery, my experience was more like a cluster of introductions and preambles resulting in a gift of unimaginable proportions: the gift of having to figure out myself, by myself.

There is a monster under your chair. There is danger in this session, and you're afraid. I have told you my story and in doing so I have littered this room with improvised explosive devices. You sit leaning in your leather chair, scared to put your feet on the floor. The concept of iatrogenic harm has you immobilized and the 799.9 deferred on Axis II was a misrepresentation of my reality. This moment has you questioning my prognosis and doubting the outcomes. I'm private pay and you have ethical standards, so you have to stay, but you're going to need a cigarette after this fifty-minute hour.

I had my initial psychotic break in the winter of 2001. I had just graduated from a high school in a small town in Ohio earlier that year. Despite an episode of grief brought about by my father's divorce from my stepmother, for which my mother took me to see a therapist, I had done well, excelling to say the least. I was president of our chapter of the National Honor Society, coeditor of the school newspaper, vice president of the student body, varsity cheerleader, a member of the ski and drama clubs, in the top ten of my class, and, eventually, the prom queen. I was flying high, not yet diagnosed as bipolar. I had not yet learned: what goes up must come down.

After my psychotic break, I returned to the same therapist. He sat in a brown leather office chair with a high back and swivel seat, twisting from desk to open area, holding his yellow legal pad and black roller-ball pen.

He had this smooth Italian accent and when he began reflecting and paraphrasing, using his basic Counseling 101 skills for empathetic listening, he sounded less empathetic with every word. Coming from him, my speech, littered with expletives, raw emotion, and grit, sounded like that of a whining, angst-ridden teen in an afterschool special. He was easily fifty years old, a child and adolescent psychologist who was excellent at treating me like a child. When he embarked on a lecture of teenage depression symptoms, I drifted off in my head.

A timepiece, a piece of time, soft rose gold brushing the thin fair hairs on my arm. I glance down at my watch; I see the time, the date: December 22, 2001, ten in the morning. I'm eighteen years old, home on Christmas break from Chicago, where I've been attending the pre-med program at Loyola University. I can smell the sweet breeze of winter and feel the crisp air against my pink frosted cheeks. In this second, I think I am well. Yet here I am, in this wacky part of town where the drug dealers live, where the meth heads hang out, where my boyfriend lives. I walk toward the paint-chipped blue duplex, twist the cold black iron knob on the door. The scent of poverty hits me just then, crack and sex smacking me in the face. My stomach sinks with doom, anticipating a crash with a looming iceberg. I know what I'm walking into. I was at the party here the night before; I know this girl probably has not left. I don't know that what is brewing in my brain is about to reach such a climax that it will take me over a decade to recall most of what will happen. I climb the stairs, creak by creak, slipping my hand across the old wood railing. Time: five minutes; number of stairs: eighteen. Had I known that I would no longer be well once I opened that old cherry door, I would have made this moment last longer.

I approach, stepping over the passed-out bodies of homeless high school runaways—mall rat Juggalos, as they call themselves. I am weaving around the pullout sofa. I arrive at the whitewashed door with no lock, no handle. If I turn around now, I will save myself. I slip my burgundy gloves off my hands and place a flat palm upon the braille-like bubbly painted door and push.

I see him, this once perfect love, this man who touched me, emotionally and physically, like I had never been touched before. He is asleep on his stomach, covered from the waist down in an orange sleeping bag. I see her, large perfect breasts heaving with each breath of sleep. I see black. I see silver. I see red. In the next few moments I find myself in a bloody fetal position in the stairwell, clutching the silver blade of a butcher knife in my raw, tear-soaked hands. I lie there and he stands over me, my wrists bleeding, his hand bleeding where I slashed it, as she walks carefully down the stairs and out the door to a neighbor's. I am still proclaiming my love to him, I am now begging for forgiveness. In this moment, I am bewitched— overtaken by a new trait, and display the ever-so-classic behavior of a borderline: I am filled with guttural, disturbing, aggressive hatred toward him, but the only thing I can say is, "Please, don't leave me."

I spent a period of unremarkable time in shock from this experience. But this transition, like each transition and transformation in my life, was built upon trauma. My inability to cope with traumas, both past and present, has made me who I am today. The idea that I would have to go backward to who I was, all while trying to move forward managing a mental illness, was traumatic in and of itself. Who I was before this psychotic break was not who I was going to be. Who I was going to be was much better, but I didn't know it at the time. I was undermedicated, then overmedicated, then unmedicated, and then self-medicated. When I finally became stable on medication that worked for me, I realized the only way to cope was to find something good out of something so terrible. I came to understand that loving and being loved would always be my downfall. I would spend the rest of my life overreacting to love, suffering from the intolerable fear, reality-based or not, that I was going to be unloved, whether today or tomorrow. So what do you do with that knowledge? You have to accept it, in order to move past it and help yourself. I found the only person that I could depend on to love me forever was me. So that is what I started working toward. It would be a long journey.

By the spring of 2002, just before my nineteenth birthday, I had filed through multiple psychiatrists. Still with the same boyfriend, I was living with four other people in a tenement apartment complex. Section 8 brought the total monthly rent down to only about sixty dollars per month, but we still couldn't pay, because all our money went to drugs. I had dropped out of college, enrolled in another university the following semester, and quickly failed out. I was refusing to live with my mother, who wanted nothing but to help me. I was cutting daily, snorting meth or anything I could find, choking down my prescribed amitriptyline one after another, and spending the rest of my time in the smoking section of the mall food court, puffing away on Camel Turkish Jade 100s. My boyfriend was still seeing the other girl, and I tolerated this, listening to the torturing stories of how happy they were, how great their sex life was, and what a waste I was—but how he still couldn't live without both of us in his life.

My second therapist positioned herself on the red velvet loveseat, propped her feet on the footstool, and popped off one shoe at a time. She had a white legal pad and a cheap Bic pen in her hand, and she asked, "You're depressed, aren't you? Do you think we should hypnotize you?"

I quickly responded, "No. It won't work; I'm not ready for that." Then an outpouring of all the reasons why I should give it a whirl spilled from her well-meaning soul. I continued to nod for the next hour, indicating understanding, but simply went on a journey to the past inside my head.

Red nylon stretches across my tan skin as I lie on the sandy beach watching the swimmers. Pure innocence pondering the enigmatic concept of love, while I twirl the blonde hair rippling down my back and soak in the sun of summer at just barely eighteen. The small-town long nights and parties at cabins in the woods and cheerleading, prom, and drama club are coming to an end. I am off to Chicago to fulfill my dreams—I have a will, there is a way, and everything is where it needs to be. Life is perfectly packaged in pink taffeta wrapping with a white satin ribbon.

So hopeful and content, thinking I need nothing more to complete my life. Something unexpected is about to show up, something that undermines everything: love, illness. Pure and utter infatuation that will rip a gaping hole in my taffeta wrapping, chew up my satin ribbon, overturn my box, and leave me empty, sick, and desolate.

Who am I to blame someone else for my illness? My boyfriend was never inside my brain, misfiring my neurotransmitters. He wasn't a chemical imbalance; he was just some guy who could have been any guy, could have been any situation, could have been nothing at all. And I still would have ended up with a mental illness. It's not helpful to ask, "What if this never happened, I never got sick?" and wish you could go back to an earlier path. Now, I can't even picture myself as a doctor. I can't picture myself as part of a traditional nuclear family. I don't remember much of the girl crowned prom queen. It's all just too boring even to think about where my life was headed. My illness was a gift; I am more creative because of it, I am more empathetic and much more capable of giving and receiving the right kind of love. This eighteen-year-old version of me could never have approached a homeless heroin addict in the street and offered to buy him a cup of coffee. She would have been terrified. The person I am today, however, would easily take his hand and sit to chat for a spell. I am able to do this now, today, in this life, all because my illness has taken me there and back.

A year after my first psychotic break, I was still with my boyfriend, living in a duplex near the Ho-Hum Motel. We were crashing in his friend's basement—well *he* was crashing in the basement; I was staying there when he wanted me, needed me, allowed me to. There was mention of starting meth production in the basement. I was so paralyzed by the substances already coursing through my veins that the details escaped me and I didn't even consider the morality or legality of the situation.

My psychiatrist at the time drove a fancy sports car. His office was littered with books, thick hardcover reference materials, and a picture of Barry Gibb. He had no legal pad, just a prescription pad. He hunched in his chair when he spoke, this soft-serve tone of voice sprinkled with, "Well, we could give it a shot," and topped with a "you can titrate up as you see fit" cherry. I didn't have the fortitude to tell him the truth: that I was a drug addict and nothing he was giving me was helping in the least. During the fifteen-minute appointment, I reflected on my current situation.

This basement, these concrete walls, the sting of methamphetamine in my nose, the burn of the tattoo gun, the pressure of the thick-gauged needle breaking my skin in every possible place; it is the pleasurable pain of anything to make me feel again. There is a sweet smell of solvent and ammonia a few feet from the mattresses laid out on the floor. I lie awake each night in this ticking time bomb, this meth lab, just to avoid my frantic fear of abandonment. Billie Holiday plays in the background, the chilling record scratching and skipping, soothing in this time of distress. I lie awake all night, running my smooth fingers up my strawberry-latticed arms, dragging them over scars, scabs, and fresh wounds. Then I run my hands across my thighs, dragging them over the bumps and bruises, some sore, some forgotten, some knotted forever in my muscles and my heart.

The only way to escape is to bump, to roll, or just to feel the catch of the rolled-up dollar bill in the hairline cracks on the cover of the Rob Zombie CD case. I will conceive my child in this basement and desecrate that gift two months later in a clinic.

As mental health professionals we push for a standard model of recovery, we push because we are told to do so—by politicians, by insurance companies, by people who research and spend careers deliberating on the best way to decrease stigma and treat illness—and we push, without a second thought on the topic, because they are the ones who pay our salaries. However, one does not need this kind of model to treat the mentally ill like human beings; providers just need a few bones of empathy—not sympathy. Empathy is a constantly confused concept in this field. You don't need to have lived my life to empathize with me; you just need to realize that I too am a human being and not my illness. I am not something to be feared, to be pitied or coddled. I'm you; we're the same.

It was March of 2003, a few weeks after my abortion. I was inconsolable. I was devastated by the choice I had made, appalled at my life, and I didn't even recognize myself. I lost my job at a fast-food restaurant because I couldn't function enough to make a cheesesteak. I ended up on Medicaid and found a community mental health agency and another psychiatrist. He was short, balding, never made eye contact. He had this thick Indian accent and dictated each session into a tape recorder. He said, "Axis one colon code two nine six period five three colon bipolar disorder most recent episode depressed comma severe without psychotic features period new line code three zero one period eight three borderline personality disorder." This was the first time I knew my diagnosis; no one in two years had ever told me. He never faced me; he faced his desk. He reviewed my ever-climbing weight and dismissed it. "You're stable on the Depakote. How are you feeling?"

The apartment bathroom, lit dimly by candles, hot steaming shower running. I look into the bathroom mirror and see a woman I don't recognize. An old woman, a hard woman, jet-black fried hair, an eyebrow ring, a tongue ring, a labret ring, an industrial ring and two solid silver hoops in her ears. There is black mascara streaming down her face, mixing and pooling with tears under her tired bleak eyes. The yellow flickering flames of the candles against the cold tile walls cast a light in the corner of her eye. She glances sideways, her dilated pupils fixed on the corner of the bathroom. The voice comes from nowhere and somewhere all at once: "You worthless piece of shit . . . you murderer . . . you're an embarrassment." Consciousness kicking in now: "What has happened to you, what have you become?"

I knew not of time; time was fleeting moments, hours, sometimes days. My memories were and are like a Goodwill puzzle, dumped across shag carpeting, half turned over, and all I can find are the corners. I wonder if the picture on the box actually matches the pieces inside. In that moment it did: both were ugly, inside and out. In that one moment, in that fire-lit bathroom, in sheer terror of what was happening in my life and in my brain—auditory hallucinations, or "voices"—I was pretty sure I was schizophrenic. I was not; I have a tendency to having psychosis when I am in a mixed-mood state. The imbalance of my medications at the time, the lack of illegal substances to self-medicate my mood, and the depression associated with my recent abortion had set off a chemical tempest. I discovered something else that day: determination.

It was an awakening. I was finally scared of myself. So scared that I went running in the opposite direction. I quickly changed everything about my situation. I dumped my boyfriend, gave up drugs, moved back home with my mom, and started school again.

Then I met him, someone I thought would fix everything that was wrong with me, the perfect, clean, sober, steady-job-holding, car-owning, football-playing, churchgoing, family-oriented, unmedicated man, Shawn.

My new therapist, a social worker, was a short blonde woman. I sat on her couch and she sat in a wooden library chair at her desk, covered in papers, disorganized. She spoke in a squeaky, high-pitched voice that was in some ways calming. "I'd like you to sign up for my group."

I obstinately quipped, "I don't do groups. Why can't we just meet one on one?" She assigned me homework; I gripped the white, freshly xeroxed copies of Wise Mind exercises from her dialectical behavioral therapy workbook and left her office. I sat outside in my green, stick-shift Saturn and wondered if therapy would really help me achieve perfection once again. Would fifty minutes and these workbook pages fix me? Would this woman be the one to bring me back to life? Or was she just another hamster stuck in the wheel that is outpatient therapy? I became lost in thought about the previous night.

I am twenty years old. Shawn and I are seated on the still, sun-warmed wooden picnic tables. Five minutes later, my life changes. I am once again addicted. His blond heroin hair sweeps across my face as we kiss for the first time, tongues slightly touching, and two old souls mesh into one tornado of passion-fueled hot cinnamon breath. I need him in my veins; he makes my face flush, my heart race, and elevates me into another dimension. I am hooked; that first taste has me forever craving his touch. I can smell him, track him like a hunter; he is my prey and I am starving for this. I need more of him, wanting to drink his soul to kill every painful moment I have ever had.

I sat night after night with my black leather tourniquet squeezing my arm, looking for anything to cut on this bright yet unreflective mirror, aching to shoot him into my veins. Throbbing in my brain because I needed to feel him, hear him, read something from him. This addiction of mine was killing us, and it tried its damnedest to kill me. The intimate relationship lasted for three years, and for two years after that I continued to chase the dragon; three years had been nothing but a taste. I couldn't let him go. He was too perfect, too normal; he was everything I used to be, he was my definition of recovery, and yet he was my relapse too. Once again, who am I to blame someone else for my illness? It was never Shawn's fault, it was never my fault; it was simply a learning experience: addiction, illness, failure, and triumph.

And there I was again. In the same situation I had so recently run away from. Addiction, this time not to drugs, but to Shawn. I appeared sane, but I was caught in the insanity of doing the same thing over and over again and expecting a different result. I'd thought this three-year period with Shawn proved that I was not mentally ill. Proved to everyone around me I was in fact recovered. But recovery is fleeting too. And it flew right out the door when Shawn left me.

My shaking body was covered in cold sweat as I sat rocking in the chair at a mental health center downtown, softly sucking in what I was sure would be my last few breaths. My body was racked with hurt, my bones and muscles sparking spasms as I clutched my knees tight to my beat-less heart. My eyes almost sealed shut with a paste of salt, I heard her call my name. She came out to greet me in the waiting room, kneeled down next to me, and said, "Come on, let's go in my office."

My first long-term psychiatrist wore catsuit-like tights, stiletto boots, and scarves, and her brown hair flowed down her back. She was thin with a slight Indian accent. Her office was quite empty and her cheap office-supply-store-brand black desk chair was simple. She put down her pen and Post-its and said, "Have you cut today?"

I said, "No."

She said, "Let me see your arms." She was smart, blunt, and honest with me.

Eventually a clean and sober mousey-brown-haired girl again, stripped of my medals and trying to find my honor, I began my journey to wellness. I got on and stayed on medications. I advocated for myself. I learned to love myself, a continued daily struggle. Six years after my initial psychotic break, I moved to Tacoma, Washington, to start a new life. However, once you stop using, you continue to crave, and thousands of miles away I relapsed on Shawn until I almost overdosed.

It has been six years and I am still itching for him. I want to scratch my pain away with anything sharp. I stand there, water pouring down on me, warm and soothing. My left hand is holding the big black kitchen knife to my throat, pushing, while my right hand presses upon the cold tile shower wall. Crying out a hard, hyperventilating moan I stand there naked, stripped of all hope. I create new track marks that night for the first time in nine years. I need the ripping feel of the serrated knife against my arm to contradict the cement sledgehammer cracking of this wall that is breaking down all around me. I put the blade to my neck once again, covered in blood, take a deep breath, and stop.

Finally, at twenty-six, one of the gifts I was able to give myself was the gift of self-control.

I have lived thirty-one years of life. For the first eighteen of those I was sane. Now I am considered "recovered." My mental illness has turned me from simple to complex, the utter definition of evolving. I am more capable now of empathy and creative thought; I have been able to develop a personal philosophy and a private relationship with a higher power. I have been able to climb the six-year mountain that was my master's degree in mental health counseling. I stopped looking to get "fixed," to "recover"; instead I adopted the attitude that I would make things work the best I could. When I accomplished that, I started looking at making things work better than I could have imagined.

My current psychiatrist, the one with the catsuit office attire and long smooth brown hair, sat across from me in her cheap office chair, which matched the one I was sitting in. As we spoke of my current strides and accomplishments, I recalled how I'd arrived at this point. I was now a case manager for the group home associated with the community mental health agency where I was still a patient . . .

I sit at my large corner desk in my bedroom at my mother's house. It's 3:00 a.m. and I'm still awake. Some habits I can't break: I'm chain-smoking at my computer, but instead of stalking my ex-boyfriend's Internet activity, I'm focusing on my own activity. I'm flipping the pages of Elizabeth Wurtzel's Prozac Nation, *where I read this word-for-word description of my own behaviors, through another woman's recollection of her own experiences. I still have access to my university's online research database and can find all the information I need there. I look for a book list on borderline personality disorder. I intend to read* I Hate You, Don't Leave Me. *I'll teach myself dialectical behavioral therapy. Better yet, I'll teach myself Zen Buddhism and cognitive behavioral therapy. I am going to eat, sleep, and breathe all I can about these illnesses in the* Diagnostic and Statistical Manual of Mental Disorders. *I am euphoric and I am manic and I am going to use this to the best of my ability until I crash into my own great depression.*

I educated myself on my illness. I made it a point to understand my symptoms and track my behaviors, learning that doing or thinking x, y, or z doesn't make me a bad person—it's just a symptom I should talk to my doctor about or investigate further. And I wrote. I had been writing since my first psychotic break; I just never realized that it was the best coping skill I had. Now, twelve years later, I have taken a basic coping skill—scribbling words into a journal—and turned it into this essay. I have gained a sense of self and self-esteem. I know more now than I ever would have without my experiences with insanity. I don't regret a single moment of illness; I accept it and learn from it, I use it every day in my life, my work, and the way I love. So no, I am not recovered. I am evolved.

I've changed offices many times, and they have always been small, covered in pictures, creative works, and books that I loan out. But the most important thing that has remained the same, over the years, is that both chairs in my office are exactly the same.

Twelve years later I sit in the other chair; it's soft and gray—ribbed corduroy that I run my nails across to feel the ripples along the tips of my fingers. The soothing repetitive motion awakens me, grounds me, allows me to accurately time the fifty-minute hour. I don't take notes (it's distracting) and I picture your story like a movie playing in my head. I try to avoid the lectures. I give silence, this cathartic silence between you and me; I am 100 percent present in your moment. I, as a person, do not exist right now. It's all about you; my empathy is grounded in you, your time, your needs, your emotions. I wait, feeling your tension and ambivalence as well as the trust rising in the room. I never had this moment for myself and I know how important it is for you.

I never had a therapist whose chair was identical to mine. It was usually tufted leather with brass coin buttons and a high back that held the power of the entire room. In this room, in these chairs, you lead and I will walk beside you as a support. I will cover my scars with my long cotton-sleeved sweater. You never need know my past. It will never inspire you, it will never lift you, and it is neither your burden nor glory to bear. My gift to you is two indistinguishable chairs.

....

Cassie Eaton has a master of science degree in mental health counseling from Walden University. She is both a peer and professional in the mental health system. She lives at home with her husband and three furry babies: Lilith Faire, Voltaire, and Sigmund Oscar.

SALVAGING PARTS

Olga-Maria Cruz

A young girl confides in her mother, "I feel schizophrenic sometimes." But only as an adult can she begin to heal the complex trauma of her childhood.

I.

I began to dissociate around the age of six. It happened at home, in the mornings when the house was quiet and I was alone in my room or in the kitchen. My consciousness would split in four pieces—most dramatically, my face seemed to split left and right. I felt each side with its own expression; I heard voices left and right as different people talking to each other. Fighting with each other.

The right side of my face was panicked and keyed up, experiencing everything I was doing (making my bed, brushing my teeth) as happening too slowly. "Hurry up! Hurry up!" it would say. "Omigod-omigod-omigod!" The left side watched the right side and scoffed. "Slow down. So what? You're so stupid. Shut up." My right face felt like my eyebrow was raised and my mouth open; on my left face, my eyebrow felt lowered, the lips pursed and curled into a sneer. I had to check my reflection in a mirror. It was curious and concerning; every time, I wondered which face would I see. Panic Face? Scorn Face? Or the Neutral Observer who floated a foot above my head? But the girl in the mirror had no expression. Her face was tenantless, affectless, which was even more frightening. I could never be sure I would come back to myself. What was left felt like a smaller version of me, withdrawn inside my chest. I was the one moving my body, but my thoughts and feelings were taken over by these strange and stronger entities.

By the time my family came around and expected me to interact, the splitting sensation would fade and my core self emerged to take over again. The episodes lasted about ten to fifteen minutes, and happened only a few times a year over the next fifteen years. But there was no way to predict or control their onset. Panic Face and Scorn Face came and went at their own will. Besides watching with a detached interest, the Neutral Observer had no distinct personality, and showed up only when Panic and Scorn started one of their fights. Other times, I didn't sense any of them at all. They did not feel like a part of me—they showed up as extreme reactions, out of proportion to what was going on. It didn't make sense to get upset about making toast or getting dressed. They even said things to each other, like "Oh my God" and "Shut up," that I would never say.

Dissociating was shocking and upsetting. At six years old I didn't have the words to make sense of my experiences. I didn't name these characters showing up in my face. I didn't talk about it, and I tried not to think about it. But a few years later, I found a way to talk to my mother. I told her, "I feel schizophrenic sometimes." I'd heard somewhere about people—crazy people—who heard voices. I explained as best I could what it felt like to have my awareness suddenly split into four pieces.

Mommy said it was okay. She didn't seem too upset, and we just let it go. No doctors or counselors were consulted, but over the years and into my twenties, whenever I had an episode, I said, "I was a little schizophrenic today," and she would say, "It's okay; you're okay." Deep down, though, I worried something was wrong. I was broken somehow, flawed. Certainly my mind, while I enjoyed using it, could not be controlled or relied on. When I learned about what was then called multiple personality disorder, I worried that Panic and Scorn might stay longer, even take over my consciousness. What happened to people with multiple personalities? What if you were just a little kid? Did you get taken away? Did you have to live in a hospital forever? I couldn't imagine growing up in a place like that—I pushed it out of my mind.

II.

Over my lifetime, I have been diagnosed with various mental conditions: major depressive disorder, generalized anxiety disorder, anorexia nervosa, post-traumatic stress disorder, seasonal affective disorder. I still suffer from each of these to some extent, but for the last two years I have been in treatment for complex trauma, which seems to be at the root of all. Post-traumatic stress disorder (PTSD) refers to the emotional response to a single terrible event—a natural disaster, a violent crime, an accident. Complex trauma, or complex PTSD, occurs when someone is exposed to multiple or repeated traumas, usually ongoing abuse or neglect, but also school or community violence, war, captivity, or the instability brought on by the loss of a parent. Most often, complex trauma originates in childhood because children are less able to escape, and so are more frequently exposed to, sequences of traumatic events. The impact of chronic trauma reaches from physical ailments to developmental difficulties to relationship disruption, emotional dysregulation, and—especially in children— dissociation.

It's not completely clear why I was dissociating so young. I have no memory of violence before age five. Certainly we moved too often; my father was absent too much; I had an insecure bond with my mother. But the greatest traumas of my life would come later. My beloved father died suddenly when I was fourteen. I was raped once and sexually assaulted at least six times, twice by strangers in parking lots, the rest by young men I was friends with or dating. The cumulative effect of all these events has been almost debilitating at times, including a surprising amount of physiological distress (headaches, irritable bowel syndrome, temporomandibular joint disorder, acid reflux, neck and back pain, fatigue) and psychic distress (chronic nightmares, anxiety and panic, depression), as well as disordered eating and disordered sleep.

I take two medications for anxiety and depression, and sit in front of a light box twice a day from October through March. I practice yoga and meditate twice a day and go to therapy every other week. What my doctor, Katie, and I do is work to connect with the pieces of my mind, to hear what they're saying and find out what they need, so we can help them integrate into my core self.

We call these pieces *Parts*. We use a variety of tools developed to heal mental trauma, within a general model called Internal Family Systems, which sees people as containing a variety of sub-personalities that work together to maintain functioning. Each of the Parts wants or needs something. Some are in distress—weeping, furious, terrified, exhausted. Others are focused, working hard to keep me on task, to keep me from feeling or even knowing about all the anger and sadness and fear that's been locked away. I shouldn't even know about their efforts; it's all supposed to be behind the scenes. But some days, for some reason, a hurting Part comes forward and shoves me in the chest or grabs me by the throat. And then I have to listen, or things get really bad. Right now, as I write this, some Part is tapping on the left side of my sternum and putting a lump in my throat. They don't want me to tell. In a few minutes, one of them will put me to sleep. I won't be able to find my words; I'll suddenly feel completely wiped out. There's only so much we can take.

Katie and I have found dozens of Parts already. The hurting ones Internal Family Systems calls Exiles. Their job is to contain negative feelings I couldn't handle when I was younger, which is why they stay young. We spent three months talking with a ten-year-old who felt completely overwhelmed by stress and abandoned by adults. There are Manager Parts, too; one that makes me faint or fall asleep when I'm overwhelmed and a Taskmaster that makes me work hard and finish what I start. There are Parts that weep and a Shaming Part that scolds them for weeping. The Shamer and Taskmaster have my mother's voice, use her words. A Part of me that wants to eat fights with the Part that wants to starve.

Some Parts have no words—they communicate via images or feelings, or physical sensations—but they all have something to say. There are Parts that hold happier memories, like a special trip to a doughnut shop, and feelings like confidence about travel and joy at being in a spotlight. Katie helps me try to soak up these positive feelings and pass them on to comfort the Exiles.

I imagine this dissociative tendency is why I never went through the anger phase of grief after my father died. I often said, "I don't really get angry." Earlier counselors found it impossible to get me to identify any of my feelings at all. I have Parts for that—Parts that hold the anger I didn't feel free to express, the fears others might scoff at, the grief I'm supposed to "be over" by now. I have Parts that secret these emotions away when I can't express or process them. Sometimes they do their jobs so well, I forget I ever had those feelings.

III.

The thing is, everybody has Parts, not just trauma survivors. Everyone experiences at least mixed feelings, and will say something like:

"Well, part of me wants to go, but part of me just wants to stay home."

"Part of me wants to trust her and part of me is shouting, *No, run away!*"

In trauma, Parts get stuck in time, and become harder to access. Hurting Parts get shut down or frozen. Protective Parts get activated. In what we now call dissociative identity disorder (DID), Parts develop not just functions but independent lives, and the core self loses time when one or another Part takes over. When I was a child, DID was one of my greatest fears. Some of my younger Parts are scared of it still. But although my dissociative experiences were scary then and can be irritating now, they are not that extreme. Katie says I am at a higher risk for DID if I were to go through another major trauma, but she also says that even DID is a wonderful, amazing coping mechanism. It would hold all the pain in different containers, and let me feel only a small amount at any one time until life got a little easier.

And everyone has experienced some level of dissociation. You zone out during a conversation; you get so tired that parts of the room seem to grow smaller or larger; you enter the world of a play, a book, or a film, and it becomes real for a brief time. Part of you knows you're you, sitting in a chair, and another part becomes a citizen of revolutionary France or Middle-earth. There is a continuum from daydreaming and suspension of disbelief to the splitting off of Parts from the consciousness and the development of other personalities. Everyone has various character elements that show up at different times, as needed. We channel our compassion when someone else is hurting, our perseverance when challenges arise.

IV.

I was fourteen when my father died suddenly of a heart attack. It was a school night, in February 1986. He had come home early from a conference to give Mommy a birthday present and left his blood-pressure medication in his hotel room. My eight-year-old brother, Cooper, and I slept through the ambulance lights and sirens, the paramedics racing into our parents' bedroom to try to resuscitate him. I woke up at 7:15 and felt there was something eerie about the house. It was spotless. My mother had been cleaning for hours, preparing for the onslaught of funeral guests. I found her furiously polishing the piano.

"Your father's dead," she said. "And you can't cry because then I'll cry and I can't cry right now. We have to go tell your brother."

So I didn't cry. My job was to help her. I was always the helper in the family, but it was clear I had to become far more adult, right away. Mommy needed me.

There was no viewing and no real ceremony—no readings, no prayers or songs. "Franklin Delano Cruz" went up on a small plaque on a mausoleum wall. We didn't even have a photo of Papí at the funeral home where we received condolences. I simply never saw him again. At the time, I was grateful to be spared the gruesome sight of his corpse. Over the years, I came to think maybe I should have been forced to see him dead. I have intense dreams, off and on, that my father is still alive. Sometimes I even need to ask my husband or my mother what is true because I wake up so terribly confused.

At first, my dreams fell into a classic pattern of denial—Papí was still alive, with us, everything just as normal. As I came to accept his death, those dreams shifted and faded. In graduate school, though, they resurfaced, with a darker twist. Papí was in the witness protection program, hiding from bad guys; he came to visit me now that I lived far from home. He felt terrible for leaving without saying good-bye.

I started dissociating more and differently after Papí died. Sometimes at the piano, I floated up to the ceiling and watched myself play. Or I floated above and behind myself as I walked down the high school corridors. In photos, I look pretty but absent, vague. That's how I felt—not completely present, because I was not complete. I felt shattered. When I felt around inside myself, I was all broken up in little pieces that had been scattered and blown far away. I knew I had to absorb the blow and pull myself back together. But I couldn't conceive of how to begin.

Mommy put me in grief counseling right away, but I didn't want to talk. All the therapists seemed awkward and dumb. They asked stupid questions: "Did you love your dad?"; "Where do you think he is right now?"; "How do you feel about that?"; "Are you angry at God for letting him die?" I just stared at the wall and wondered how they ever earned those fancy diplomas. My father was dead; he was in a jar because he was just ashes now, and obviously it felt really, really bad. Who would be happy? And he wasn't my "dad," he was *Papí*. But the counselors didn't deserve to know that. How could they ask me "did" I love him? I *do* love him. Do, do, do, do, do. I wasn't angry—I was just so, so sad. I was so sad I couldn't talk. I didn't have words. I could barely move. One counselor said I needed to cry. He would contact my school to make sure I had a quiet place and permission to leave class.

Mom thought that was bullshit. "When you're at school, you need to focus on school." So I never let myself cry there, either.

Mom went to counseling, too. She had started having panic attacks, though she didn't tell me about it, and the term *panic attack* wasn't yet in our vocabulary. All I knew was she had trouble driving and had to keep the windows down and the heater off so she could concentrate. Cooper and I shivered with the winter wind in our faces and stayed very quiet. One night, a few weeks after the funeral, Mommy walked out of the house and drove away, without saying good-bye, without saying where she was going or when she'd be back. Coop and I looked at each other. What if she *didn't* come back?

"It'll be okay," I told him. "I'll take care of you." I thought for a minute. What could we do, really? I was only fourteen. "We could go and live with Aunt Kathy." Mom's sister lived in Oregon and never visited us. We kept looking at each other, tacitly understanding. Mommy would probably come back, and in a few hours, she did. But Cooper and I knew we had to be extra good. We had to keep her. We would stop bickering, do more chores. We wouldn't ask for anything. I would try harder to act cheerful.

She'd tried before and failed, but Mommy stopped smoking for good the day Papí died, and I started abusing painkillers. Nothing illegal, just over-the-counter meds: Tylenol, ibuprofen, and something called Percogesic. The package said, "For enhanced relief of pain." I started taking double and triple the adult dose.

Sometimes my body would numb itself with no help from me. I slept a lot in the afternoons. I fainted quite a few times, especially when I had some extra stressor in my life or forgot to eat. I was especially disconnected from my body at that point, and just not in touch with my hunger. When I did eat, nothing tasted good.

. . .

V.

All the napping and fainting and numbing was part of a very strong and natural trauma response called hypo-arousal. The fight-or-flight response is hyper-arousal, where adrenaline floods the nervous system: the heart races, the legs might shake, palms sweat, head pounds. But the "fight" and "flight" options are useful only when the body can move and there is a chance of escape. When trauma is inescapable, the nervous system has another strategy—to freeze. In hypo-arousal, the adrenaline needed for fighting or fleeing is shut off; the body is immobilized or numbed as emotional and cognitive functions are disrupted. Of these situations, trauma survivors say things like, "I couldn't move"; "I couldn't think"; "My heart stopped"; "I couldn't breathe"; "I thought I was going to pass out."

Memories of episodes of hyper-arousal tend to be strong and vivid; memories of episodes of hypo-arousal tend to be foggy or nonexistent. For me, hypo-arousal occurs when I get overwhelmed. My mind feels foggy and goes blank; my breath gets shallow; I start to feel like I'm going to fall asleep. When it happens in counseling, Katie talks to me, helps me come back to a more neutral place so I can stay present. I struggled with hypo-arousal after my father's death because my body-mind was overwhelmed with shock and grief. I didn't want to be alive. If my family hadn't needed me or if I hadn't felt they did, I would absolutely have ended my life. As it was, I did try once.

VI.

It was the night before I was to take the SAT. I must have been sixteen, but inside, I felt exactly the same as I had in February 1986. My grief hadn't resolved at all. I still felt that life without my father, life in a universe where beloved fathers could disappear overnight, was not worth slogging through. I was under a tremendous amount of pressure at school, mostly from teachers who wanted me to perform feats of academic brilliance on the SAT. Walking down the halls, I was exhorted by various teachers leaning out their classroom doors:

"Olga-Maria! You working on your math?"

"Olga-Maria? How's that math coming along?"

Already a bit of a perfectionist and deeply aware since the fourth grade (long division) and fifth grade (fractions) that math was not my strong suit, I was embarrassed that other people, grown-ups, teachers, were expecting some sort of huge leap of progress from me—on one Saturday morning, on a national exam. What if I choked?

I didn't want to let anyone down. I *really* didn't want to let myself down. I had to be amazing. In my mind, I was competing not against my current classmates but against the superstars of the best schools in the country. And, with Papí gone, I needed all the scholarship money I could get. It was too much to face. I took a whole bottle of Percogesic before bed. I didn't leave a note.

Percogesic bottles are particularly small. I was disappointed to wake up the next morning and disconcerted to find my eyes not working at all. I switched on the lights but saw only darkness. Trying not to panic, I pulled off my clothes, turned on the shower, blind, and then collapsed on the floor. My mother heard me fall, came in, and pulled me so that my head was lower than my heart. She turned the shower all the way to cold and held my upper body under the water. I came to again, gasping. No SAT for me that day.

Percogesic is essentially Tylenol plus Benadryl, an antihistamine with strong sedative properties. Side effects include low blood sugar, which leads to fatigue, drowsiness, dizziness, fainting, and, at high doses, blurred vision. It took a few hours for my eyesight to return, longer for my mother to recover from the worst moment of her life, those ten or so minutes when she thought her daughter had killed herself. Longer for me to understand how important I was to her, and to forgive myself for putting her through that. We moved forward, carefully, treating each other more gently and with gratitude. We said, "I love you," more frequently. I promised myself I would try harder, try not to worry her. I would stay alive for her and for Cooper.

VII.

It took another fourteen years for me to begin to feel whole. I went to two counselors in high school, four in college, and three in grad school—trying to find someone who could help me not want to die, help me want to eat, want to be sexual. Healing from childhood trauma takes time. And trauma survivors are extra vulnerable to predation, like prey animals with a limp, or an eye missing. Through childhood, adolescence, and young adulthood, I suffered numerous sexual assaults. We're still sifting through those memories and aftereffects, which include depression, anxiety, anorexia. All the disorders and conditions previous counselors diagnosed and tried to treat stem from trauma. So too the dissociation, frequent fluctuation between hyper- and hypo-arousal, overall numbness, low sex drive, the clumsiness that leaves me with frequent bruises on my knees and elbows. I wanted to be well. But only an adult can heal a child's pain. I had to grow up in order to be fully capable of addressing the damage done to my younger psyche, and I needed a trauma specialist.

• • •

When I visit Katie she'll ask me what's on my mind, and then I scan my body for uncomfortable sensations. Often there's a pressure or gripping feeling in my chest or stomach. If I breathe into the discomfort and mentally send some compassion, the pain will often shift. We follow the sensation wherever it leads while Katie helps me maintain a gratitude for the Part who is coming forward, for its willingness to communicate.

It helps to have either a headset with music that moves from the left ear to the right, or to hold paddles that vibrate back and forth. The right-to-left-to-right motion imitates the rapid movement of our eyes during the dreaming phase of sleep. The music especially soothes my Parts and helps calm their physical manifestations. I also find it helps me drop into the awareness of whatever Part has come forward. I've done some work as an actor, and getting in touch with a Part involves the same inner mechanisms I would use to find past emotions and memories in order to embody a character: it requires simultaneous relaxation and concentration, a radical openness. An actor must respect and love her character even if that character says or does horrible things. Perhaps her first task is to find compassion for her character. Every Part needs compassion, even if it has been creating an addiction or giving you headaches, or night terrors, or indigestion. Most of my Parts are young, some even pre-verbal. A lot of what they need is security, love, for their feelings to be validated, and reassurance that things are better now, that the trauma is over and we are safe.

Katie will prompt me with questions for whoever is present: How old are you? Where are you right now? Can the Part feel my presence? What does she need from me? What does she want me to know? As the conversation progresses, sensations will move and shift, sometimes dramatically. A Part might be worked up and hyper-aroused, with a flushed face, a louder voice, and a pounding heart. More often, we run into hypo-arousal as a Part's defense mechanism against our efforts to uncover strong negative emotions. I try to remind the troubled Part that she has me, and Katie, and my husband and our dog as constant resources, and she also has the whole network of other Parts. If one Part needs to cry or throw a fit, another can take over for a while.

One friend I've told about this work said it's as if I were a haunted place, and my counseling sessions were séances. Like ghosts, the Parts can be disruptive and inconvenient. Often they come forward when I'm feeling relaxed and comfortable, which makes sense psychologically—we are better able to deal with traumatic memories and the aftereffects of traumatic events when we're feeling stronger—but I don't *want* to be choked with grief in the middle of a yoga class. I have a hard time falling asleep without Parts rising up, looking for connection. Most nights I try to lose myself in a novel or a movie, someone else's story.

VIII.

The more I try to write and the darker the memories are that I retrieve, the more resistance I find from certain Parts. This week it was a Protector I call Sarabeth, who keeps me from thinking about upsetting memories, usually by distracting me with song lyrics. I first encountered Sarabeth as I was trying to write about two incidents of sexual assault that happened when I was in college. Every time I went to those memories, my head would fill with songs like a jukebox stuck on repeat.

Working with Katie, I learned that Sarabeth is fourteen years old—she came into being to keep me from thinking about my father in the weeks and months after his death. She is amazingly strong and diligent. I need to ask Sarabeth's permission every day before I can write about certain traumas. For some people, I imagine, writing is therapeutic. For me, the writing is just hard— mentally and emotionally. Only by doing the work of therapy am I able to attempt to find words for my experiences; Katie not only teaches me psychological terms, she helps me uncover images and metaphors to understand my younger selves, their burdens, and their longings.

In talking to Sarabeth, we couldn't just jump right into the memories she blocks. We began by getting to know her and building a rapport, so that she could learn to trust us and open up little by little. Katie says some Parts want to release feeling, but Sarabeth holds only a vague sense of sadness, and a deep exhaustion, which manifests as the sound of a low, droning bass line. We asked Sarabeth if she'd like some sort of support to come into her life—a friend, an ancestor, an animal, a place, a spiritual being. She knows exactly what she needs. She wants to stand in a field, surrounded by trees and filled with sunlight: a soft, golden light, sparkling, moving up as well as down, lifting as well as enlightening. In Sarabeth's vision, the light makes everything more spacious and open—it creates more space between the trees and cleaner air to breathe. In her vision, the light has a sparkling sound, like harps and bells. It breaks up the heavy bass line of her sadness and fatigue. She can see for miles around, and there are mountains on the horizon. There are places she can go, but Sarabeth doesn't want to *have* to go anywhere. She wants light and space and peace and freedom. She wants a rest, and I know I can use my imagination to help her. I will keep telling her that everything will be okay if she relaxes for a while. I will find that sort of space in my own life and send its quiet beauty in her direction. I will try to get her to that meadow.

....

Olga-Maria Cruz, PhD, writes and teaches in Louisville, Kentucky. Her poems have appeared in Poetry East, Ars Intepres, *and the* Chaffin Journal, *among others. She is completing a memoir of trauma and recovery with support from the Kentucky Foundation for Women and the Kentucky Arts Council.*

HITBODEDUT

Catherine Klatzker

A woman struggles with alternate identities she's never acknowledged out loud. With encouragement from her therapist, Dr. D., she heads off to a silent residential retreat; in the woods, she has a startling breakthrough.

Watching my alternate identities, my "Parts," was like watching snow melt—more listening than seeing except for the puddles. Like the crunch of ice sheets sliding off a roof, their sudden eruptions jolted me. I cringed. As an adult living in sunny warm Los Angeles, parts of me were frozen in time. As a child, when I had glimpsed Good Daddy changing into Bad Daddy, my Parts came to the rescue. I didn't have to be present or know what happened. My Parts held those moments until they began thawing, leaking, eight years ago when I was fifty-four. I was beginning to believe my voices and my memory, which was still piecemeal and fragmented. Yet, even as I sensed what was true, I wondered what was real.

I visited Dad in Northern California for over five years after my mother's death. He was constipated, arthritic. He had a very slow-healing vascular leg ulcer, a slow-growing prostate cancer, and his knees gave out when he tried to stand. He lost a little weight, hovering below three hundred pounds for the first time in many years. He was ninety-two years old. After Thanksgiving, he agreed to enter the hospital for his constipation and to get some X-rays. He understood he might not be released unless he could stand up on his own. I wondered if he intended to apply himself to physical therapy or whether he was resigned to his impending death.

At the end of December, he was moved to a skilled-nursing facility in Danville. I felt compelled to continue visiting him, hoping for some acknowledgement of what I increasingly knew was true.

"Catherine, if there's anything you ever want to say to your father while he's alive, now is the time," my therapist, Dr. D., said. While his statement was true, it was also true that I clenched with unbelievable fear in his presence. Subtle triggers from my dad sent alarms activating my alternate identities, my Parts, and freeze, flight, and fright reactions vied for control before I dissociated altogether.

To dissociate means to detach, separate, disconnect. A person with a dissociative disorder experiences a disconnection and lack of continuity between thoughts, memories, surroundings, actions, and identity. Symptoms range from amnesia to alternate identities. Sometimes I "went away" or spaced out unpredictably, and sometimes other Parts took over for me, which I tried to overlook. I didn't think of my Parts as dissociated identities because I dissociated *that* thought as well. Essentially, I dissociated from my dissociation. It was all very circular and very confusing.

After spending five hours with my dad one day in January, I realized how much difficulty I had staying present with him, not dissociating when he looked at me, when he raised his voice, when he ruminated on his life. Nevertheless, I felt like we needed to break Dad's rule of silence. Sometime soon I needed to say what could never be said before.

He was still in the nursing facility in March 2008 when I went to a residential Jewish meditation retreat in Mill Valley, California, not far from Danville. Silent residential retreats are an opportunity for intensive meditation, like an immersion course in a language. Meditating at home, I found that staying present and mindful in a silent setting rewarded me with flashes of insight and feelings of deep gratitude and stillness. I hoped an extended retreat would help me to find some clarity and balance.

In a therapy session before I left, I wondered if I was ready for the lengthier retreat. "You're strong enough now," Dr. D. said. He knew the risk of lengthy retreats. In the past, I had been overcome by my fallback dissociation; I had spaced out and "gone away" in trance states that were the opposite of my mindfulness practice. Now he thought I could stay present without drifting off into a terrorized, fragmented state.

"You're stronger," Dr. D. said. He wouldn't let me drift off or sink into the cringing, exploding, pulverizing sensations of helplessness that I could only describe as "fragmenting." He told me he would protect all of us, the many unknown parts that held me together.

My lip quivered as I realized that Dr. D. really saw me. For the first time he invited all of us into the room to speak to him, the "whole family." We had never even said *dissociative identity disorder* (DID), and we didn't now. I barely said it to myself. I knew I heard from, and talked to, distinctive and separate Parts of myself; I had even written about them by name for some time. Yet I clung to my belief that my Parts were not actually dissociated identities because I lived a normal life. *I was normal*, not insane. I compartmentalized my Parts from DID. Every time the thought came up, it fled.

Dr. D. had so far spoken only of a generic inner child, not the child Parts I experienced, and I hadn't corrected him. People have conflicting needs and wants, heart versus mind and ego versus id—conflicts of desires and impulses. He worked with me to move toward a greater coherence. His "method" was to be as receptive as possible while not imposing a particular theory or diagnostic structure. All the same, I was afraid of his diagnosis if he found out my Parts were real, if he were to tell me they were alters of a dissociative disorder, so it remained unsaid.

Only one day into the weeklong retreat, I was critical and full of internal suggestions for running a better operation. I had been coordinating one-day mindfulness meditation retreats for professional health caregivers for over three years. As an organizer, I was disgruntled with my first day in Mill Valley. I intellectualized and distanced myself from deeper explorations. After one night of my negative energy, my roommate abruptly moved out of our shared room into the larger, crowded dorm upstairs, and I turned my disparagement on myself in haiku.

> *Bone with no marrow*
> *Where is the heartfelt practice?*
> *Is it them, or me?*

In the morning at the time for the silent Amidah, I cynically wondered what Rabbi Roth, the retreat leader, could possibly have to say, since I was sure every single participant already knew the Amidah, the central prayer in each of the daily services, said silently and standing. I strained to hear his soft-spoken voice when he announced, "I want to suggest a practice of *hitbodedut* for Amidah this morning, of walking out into the wilderness around our grounds here and speaking out loud, *not* silently, to God from your heart. The way people do this is to go off alone where no one can hear you and say what comes up for you, what you yearn for. Reach into your heart and speak out loud to God. Some people offer up their own words of gratitude. Some people get mad and yell at God. It's your heart. Just speak."

Deeply skeptical, I walked out among the redwoods. I started tentatively, talking to myself.

"God is a construct, a transitional object, a cultural transitional phenomenon." I was intellectualizing again, talking myself out of the whole enterprise. After a lifetime of trying to talk to God, I'd finally begun to suspect I was talking to myself. "God is a verb," I said. "My mind is a verb, everything is process and *hineni*, here I am. Anyway, God is not the name, there is no name." I was rambling, and I knew it. I paused and studied a giant tree that towered nearby.

I took three steps backward and three steps forward, and then I stood with my feet together and surrendered to the moment. "Dear God, I want to find my little girl, to know her, to know where she went when she went away, and why. I need to be whole. I want to matter." Suddenly, I felt a yearning for life to matter and deep agonizing gasps escaped my throat. "My life is empty, I cannot find my selves, and I do not matter at all."

Something was happening. Without warning, all of me and every Part cried out like a wounded animal or a child taking great jagged, heaving gulps of air. A wild fox sauntered down the path to investigate. All my Parts were out. All of us stared down the fox. We looked each other in the eye, each of us fearless. The fox, smaller than I would have expected, had I expected a fox at all, turned around and walked back up the path. My fearlessness felt pulled, as if by a cord, after the departing fox. Both fear and fearlessness competed inside me; my alter Cat was out. Great wailing sobs spewed from deep down, past my throat. My alter Tina sank deeper into the reality of "not mattering." Baby and Cathie came into blurry focus, and I doubled over with the weight of their felt experience. I had never before felt all my Parts together at the same time.

I'd never come to terms with their creation in my childhood, an existential choice I didn't know I'd made, and I'd done my best *not* to know it: how they'd been hatched whole and complete and named so long ago. The traumatic memories I'd avoided for so many decades could not be safely approached without first overcoming my fear of dissociative Parts: a chasm opened up, they were all there, shifting in and out of each other, none of us avoiding each other, smack in the midst of everyone's experience of fear, anger, open-heartedness, disbelief, pain, worthlessness, longing, disgust, innocence, and more pain. Cat and Tina and Katie, normally so protective, were no match for the flood that burst through that fissure.

My child-self had been quieted for decades. She cried this hard only when terrible things were done to her. My full-blown sensory memory took me back to that time. Her fear wound itself around my neck and throat. *I* had never cried for those things. Maybe Baby had, but I hadn't. Now, I felt her helplessness. I noticed Cathie guarding my head with my arms, and I felt the first assault of genital sensations. *No!* It felt like body memory. Many child-selves were present, fully formed and named, yet Cathie was the pivotal Part I kept returning to. I felt a fear bordering on terror as I shielded my head and tried to fold my body over to make my middle inaccessible. Shame flooded through me and confirmed that Cathie's frenzy came from other invasions that had taught her what to expect. These other selves, these Parts, seemed separate, but they were me. Yet they were not me. What happened to them was happening to me right now. So far, my Parts could only talk to me in my body. This was my most profound experience of their communication by sensory reenactment.

I knew I usually left Cathie and the others alone in trauma at the same time I knew I was left alone. Leaving them was identical to leaving myself, to dissociating. That knowledge, that when I had dissociated and "gone away" I had split apart and left her to this dread, to unnamed violations, and to this terror—both me and not-me—made me feel, as I crouched now among the trees, like I was breaking. The only way to hold myself together was to embrace Cathie tightly, so I wrapped my arms around myself hard and rocked her. The rest of me slowly came back together. I felt like I couldn't stop crying. Ever. My heart hurt, my neck hurt, my groin hurt, and none of this should have been happening, should have ever happened to her, to *me*. When my body was bent over and my tears flooded the forest floor, my consciousness blipped—a hiccup in a time warp—*it's me, it's not me, it's me, it's not me*—I didn't want to push Cathie away anymore. I only wanted to hold her.

Back at the retreat house, the aftermath of body memory settled into *just this breath, no judgment, just this moment,* and meditation sustained me for the rest of the day, but the floodgates of crying reopened when I was alone in my room. A condition of dissociative disorders is that visceral flashbacks are often triggered by emotional overload. I didn't know that then; I believed my feelings could overwhelm and destroy me. Even though it was a silent retreat, I left Dr. D. a voice mail that night. In six years of therapy, he had never seen or heard me cry. He voice-mailed back: "I am sending wishes for your safety and healing. Crying is a wonderful way of opening your heart and cleansing your wounds. It is scary, but you seem ready for it. Talking to someone can help keep you feeling safe and grounded."

When Dr. D. and I connected the next day, I assured him that hearing his voice had made me feel more secure. His call was a touchstone to get me through the days ahead.

During the morning's first meditation, the inner voices said, "I couldn't protect you." I understood these were protective Parts, Cat and Tina together, and I was deeply touched. "I couldn't protect you," Cat repeated. She wanted me to understand how hard my Parts had worked for over fifty years to protect me. My Parts all came out in full force at my invitation in Mill Valley where *we* felt safe. They seemed to be telling me body-details of childhood terror, of things they had protected me from knowing until now. I still spun into denial that my Parts were dissociative identities. I knew they were aspects of me and also separate. I could not wrap my mind around me, Catherine, actually being a multiple. I couldn't do it because I disconnected from the thought each time it came up.

> *Window behind me*
> *I stare blankly through the room*
> *The tulip opens*

I discovered a roughhewn stairway down to a landing with a little bridge above a pond. When I went there and sat with Cathie and Baby, great sobs escaped from my depths, from a long deferred self who was vulnerable, completely open, delicate. I was alone. I was sure if anyone stumbled on my place, they would look away and give me my privacy. We were safe. Opening to this sweet, tender child-self initiated an emotional reenactment of old pre-verbal trauma. I thought deeply about this. I felt a connection to others who might have had no protectors, and I imagined their faceless presence around me. In the woods, I talked and I kept talking. Afterward I didn't know what I had said, what *we* had said—it was blank mostly—but it felt like a healing ritual that I needed very much.

The yearning quality of talking to God in nature allowed my tender young voice expression, allowed her to cry out, and I knew I'd have to sit with her terror and helplessness for a while. I had been so afraid of my Parts, their pain and their history—even phobic, and I never expected their grace, or their courage, or their extraordinary sweetness. I didn't expect to find such innocence, to be so drawn to deeply knowing my own Parts.

I'm happy to say
It's still raining in the woods
Stairs go down and up

In the next days, during services, I walked again and again
to the woods to talk and cry deeply, crying "no-no-no-no-no,"
my hands and arms shielding my head, my body bent over, nose
dripping and my tears soaking the ground. The vaginal sensations
unmistakably informed me that something had happened that I
didn't want to remember. It was no longer so easy to "go away"
from my body. Meditation was my training ground for allowing
body memory. Staying neutral, suspending beliefs, sitting with
each moment, was a mighty practice. Mindfulness allowed me to
stay present.

Dissociative disorders, above all, interfere with being present,
and I had a variety of ways to avoid the world. Before meditation
taught me to be present in my life, I would dissociate and Baby
would come and hold my panic without my knowledge. Cathie
and Katie and Tina and Cat would continue to protectively
hold my history out of memory, and it would continue to leak
irregularly into my life like a resistant virus. There had been
some level of seemingly random terror in my body since infancy,
relieved by the dissociative activities of spacing out, amnesia, self-
harm, and cutting myself.

Hitbodedut took me totally by surprise. In Mill Valley I found
and claimed my Parts. I recognized an innocence, a sweetness and
fragility in the little girl I spoke to, whom I loved the way one loves
a newborn—fiercely, and I promised I would never leave her.

When it was time to leave after the retreat, I kept turning
around and walking back into the woods until I ultimately forced
myself to get in my PT Cruiser and drive away. I felt like a mother

unable to leave her daughter's body, imagining her cold and alone, going back to her over and over. One of the governing rules I discovered in the physics of my alternate Parts was that they consistently seemed external to me—outside—even though they spoke to me from inside myself. It wasn't logical, but I felt that I was leaving a key part of myself in the redwoods. I felt unsteady when I left.

I went directly to confront my father.

It was an easy drive to his Danville skilled-nursing facility. I still hoped for what he would not give. *Maybe he'll apologize for all the harm he's done. Maybe he'll concede the truth and be sorry.* But he didn't seem like the same man who had hurt me as a child. I hardly knew him. He was unhappy, grumpy, and sad. He sagged weakly in his hospital bed. He had been refusing physical therapy. His skin hung off his frame. He was uncomfortable, and he slept poorly. I brought him some hot coffee from Starbucks. He ate a little yogurt for me.

I'd always wanted a protector. Now I was past that. I wanted acknowledgment, maybe some remorse, but Dad had said everything he wanted to say. He would never acknowledge any wrongdoing, any trespass or betrayal, certainly nothing that he had done when he'd been drinking. When I attempted to say something, Dad shut his eyes against me. I wanted proof, *dammit*, because I had a built-in denial network that got tripped by a nuance of speech, by a glance, by silence. Facing him, I was ready to believe I was totally wrong, that he was kindness itself—he looked so helpless—that he was somehow not my perpetrator. My alter Katie was out and we sat quietly as Dad drifted off to sleep. She had always kept me from knowing there had been no trustworthy adult in my life. Katie expected to find Good Daddy when the survival value of that was long past. I didn't know Katie well enough yet to counsel her, *This is where you used to try to make him into Good Daddy. I see how much we needed that. You can ease up now.*

It was a semi-tranquil time together. His presence still paralyzed me even when my body was filled with felt evidence. I didn't feel real in his presence unless he said I was. And he didn't. He took so much of me away from me. The assault of my body memories and my own child memory accused and condemned my father before I walked into his room, and I went speechless. I was no one again, invisible. When I tried to confront my father, my voice froze.

Inside, my Parts agitated. I did not feel angry; Cat carried my anger. I did not hate Dad in those moments. Cathie and Tina and Baby hated him, and I agreed with them, but I didn't feel it. I wanted to be held. So did they. As my father slept, I was the mute ghost that sat next to him in his room, stubbornly waiting for some acknowledgment before his death.

Looking back, I sometimes think a better person might have found some peace then and let the past go. I was not that person. I was not any singular person; it didn't feel like a solo decision to move on when I had Parts still bringing *our* past into my present, releasing unrelenting body memories. I didn't quite grasp the conflict that twisted me into helplessness in his presence, the inherent contradiction between, on the one hand, understanding my protector's unthinkable betrayal, stripping me of his protection, and, on the other, Katie's simultaneous devotion to Dad. Katie adored Daddy. My only proof was my life.

On the long drive home to Los Angeles I obsessed about the vulnerability of my childhood. I listened to music, a 2004 CD of David Zeller's psalms of yearning for protection and shelter, and I cried all the way back to LA. I felt hesitant to enter my condo without first seeing Dr. D. and finding some courage. I was filled with a sense of imminent loss, that my intimacy with my child Parts would be lost to me when my life returned to normal. I sped down the I-5 crying at the thought of losing my delicate innermost Parts. Then I thought, *Who protected me?*

. . .

My speech was frenzied, my hands were shaky, and I felt a little crazed when I buzzed into Dr. D.'s office on my way home. At the best of times, bringing reawakened awareness from silent retreats back into community is jarring. It is, in fact, a re-entry from a rarified world. Dr. D. was hosting my re-entry, and I was suddenly ashamed. The world was too real; I felt unreal and less than sane. Leaning back in his chair, his feet propped up on the gray leather ottoman, Dr. D. seemed curious as he inquired about the location of my body memories and asked me to notice details of what had been an emotional flood.

Details. Physical details like holding my hands over my head and face, doubling over . . . I went mute. I felt my Parts backing off. I suddenly could not mention the vivid re-experiencing of jostling and prodding, my horror and grief, my child's tactile memory. I had voices inside arguing that it couldn't mean what I thought, answered by a voice that said *something is happening, stop*, and another that said *no no no*, and another that said *this is not happening, it is not real*, and I was deeply ashamed of noticing my vagina so much, let alone talking about it to this man who had never spoken directly to my Parts. I could not tell him about switching in and out of *me, not me, me, not me*. How could I tell him I was dirty and dissociating?

Dr. D. saw my confusion. "Who is here?" he asked.

His question interrupted my Parts, and I was annoyed. Safety was always my priority, and all my Parts had to feel safe with Dr. D., not just my primary self. I trusted Dr. D., but my Parts didn't. Shame resurfaced, and I struggled to speak.

"When I talked out loud in the woods, something broke open in me," I said. "This child Part is fragile and dear to me, and I'm afraid to lose her when I go home."

Now, in retrospect, it seems a strange concern, given what had just opened up. I was leaving out half of my story. *I had claimed my Parts.* It was a monumental breakthrough, but at the time, my entire perspective was from inside the storm of that misgiving. I could not see my way past the fear of losing Cathie and the others.

"We all do the best we can," Dr. D. said, and I thought he was speaking to my Parts, not to me.

"You're comforting my protectors." I said *protectors* as a euphemism for my Parts and I held my breath, observing his response. I had studiously hidden my fear of DID, the distress and horror of suspecting multiple identities.

"Yes," he acknowledged. It was possible he was speaking of an internal protective ego mechanism, a conscious protective device, a mental trick. But it seemed to me he was speaking of my particular Parts for the first time. Dr. D. had noticed shifts in my consciousness and his own shifts in response to my experience. My eye movements, body language, and speech weren't congruent with speaking to one person. When he asked me about the shifts he was observing—*What's happening? Who's here?*—I was always vague and deliberately misleading. He tracked my experience and tried not to get ahead of me.

I seemed to Dr. D. to be accessing other emotional states, unconscious emotional aspects alongside and parallel with mine. *This is different,* he noted to himself and later told me. The nuances of separation he observed with me were vastly different than what he experienced with other clients. I didn't appear afraid, yet I seemed to be reporting on a fear communicated to me by someone else. *Whose fear was it?* It was like someone was talking to me, and I was the interpreter for Dr. D. He tells me now that he thought, *What is it you're accessing that's afraid?* So he spoke to *all* of me, the *whole* Catherine, without knowing there were separate identities within.

I listened as myself and also from the perspectives of my Parts as Dr. D. spoke to all my Parts, and this moved me. Cat and Tina and all the others—they were there.

"I need you to talk me through going home," I finally said. "I'm just so afraid I'll be leaving her again . . ." My chin started to tremble, my teeth to chatter, like when it's cold outside. The shivering felt foreign, from another Part of me, and I inquired within myself, *who is this?* "I know I've left her before, and I'm not leaving her now, but I still feel afraid of losing her." I willed the trembling to stop.

"Catherine, she has been a part of you since her beginning, and she will always be with you. You can put up walls, but she is always a part of you," Dr. D. said. He seemed very sure of himself. Before I left, we made an appointment for the next day and another for later in the week.

I knew that two distinct processes were underway: the opening to my sweet child Part and the emotional reactivation of old trauma. My memories were locked in alternate identities, out of reach until now, and I had no operating manual for how that worked. So far I hadn't figured out that the only way my Parts would communicate was by re-experiencing, or sensory reenactment, another critical law of my dissociative disorder.

It was a first thaw, a turning point foreshadowing an eventual integration of Parts that was painfully slow for many more years until it wasn't, as deceptive as watching snow melt. It's easy to miss the tiny buds of wildflowers on the prairie under the slush from so many fierce winters.

Wholeness was my goal. I wanted freedom from breaking apart and disappearing and losing entire chunks of my life. Freedom from the terror. When I was deeply in the healing process, I would unconsciously begin to integrate. For me, this was a process, not an event. Parts didn't go away and suddenly leave me alone. Dr. D. was right: I couldn't lose them if I wanted to. Instead, I learned to become a home for my Parts, which has allowed the possibility of a unified identity. The day would come that all my inner partitions would come down and the qualities, memories, and feelings of my Parts would no longer be separate. They would be me.

....

Catherine Klatzker's work may be seen in Emrys Journal *and in the* Intima: A Journal of Narrative Medicine. *She was a Ragdale Foundation writing resident and her work won the 2014 nonfiction prize from* Tiferet Journal. *"Hitbodedut" is adapted from her memoir-in-progress. Catherine is a recently retired pediatric ICU RN and for ten years she has coordinated mindfulness retreats for professional health caregivers coping with death.*

LIVE A LITTLE

Ellen Holtzman

A therapist struggles to help Ann, a patient suffering from tremendous anxiety. When Ann doesn't respond to cognitive therapy, however, the author reminds herself that good care requires flexibility: "In the dance of therapy, she leads, I follow."

Ann sits down in my office, visibly short of breath. Dark hair frames a pale face made ashen by the black glasses she wears. She has the sweet voice of a young girl, but Ann is forty years old. "I can't drive. I can't work. I can barely leave the house," she tells me, avoiding my gaze. Her chest moves quickly up and down.

My heart beats fast, mirroring Ann's unease. As she fidgets in her seat, I imperceptibly—at least I hope imperceptibly—shift my body to get comfortable again. *Get a grip*, I say to myself. *I am a psychologist, and I am supposed to be helping Ann.* But her agitation is contagious. Prone to anxiety myself, I am getting more and more nervous with each passing minute.

Glancing around my office, I try to compose my emotions. A large window fills the room with sunlight, making the office warm and cozy. I study the chair I always offer to patients, including Ann. This navy-blue chair is soft and plush, reminding me of the chair in my parents' home where I curled up as a young girl, worried and shy, listening to the rain against the window. I have lost count of the number of patients who affectionately call it the "comfy chair."

Perched stiffly on the edge of the comfy chair, Ann can see a framed 1970s poster advertising *QE2* cruises. "To the Caribbean, Europe, Around the World," the poster says. "For Once in Your Life, Live!"

I stumbled upon the print at a yard sale and hung it in my office because its blue background matched the navy comfy chair. As the years have passed, I have become increasingly fond of this picture. I look at it and think back to my twenty-year-old self on my first solo European trip, my confidence growing with each new city I explored. But Ann's background turns out to be very different from my own easy childhood. Observing her vacant stare, I am certain the poster's message means nothing to her. She looks like a woman who is unable to live, even a little.

She quickly launches into her story. "I was fine until I gave up the drugs—alcohol, pot, cocaine, Ecstasy." Her tone is matter-of-fact, as if she were reciting a grocery list.

The drugs have controlled her life since she was twelve. Ecstasy was her best, total love. "It is as if you are feeling the love you might have for your newborn baby," she says as she rocks her imaginary infant in the cradle her crossed arms form. "But a million times better," she adds softly.

Drugs are expensive, and Ann lies to her boyfriend, Tom, about where all her money has gone. "Daily expenses," she says to him as nonchalantly as she possibly can when he asks why they have so little money.

Watching a television show about the benefits of honesty and fearful that Tom is about to leave her, Ann finally confesses her drug addiction. To her surprise, he says, "We are a family together, and everything will be okay."

Free of the secrecy and shame of her drug habit, she discovers that the next few days are the happiest in her life. Tom loves her, and she feels hopeful about the future. Ann gives up drugs.

Soon after, she gets in her car. She is supposed to visit her dad who has seriously injured himself driving drunk. Ann dislikes her dad and doesn't want to see him. She thinks of this trip as an obligation she would prefer to avoid.

Driving to her dad's, she feels lightheaded, short of breath. She inhales, but she can't seem to get enough air. Her chest grows tight and painful. Her heart is pounding. Terrified and gasping, Ann pulls her car over to the shoulder of the highway, turns around, and heads home. "I must be having a heart attack," she tells herself.

Around the same time, her employer moves her to another office, requiring a longer, more traffic-filled commute. The drive back and forth to work torments her. She is terrified that she will not be able to breathe every time she gets into the car. One day she decides that she cannot face the drive, and she makes an appointment with her doctor.

Soon she is diagnosed with a panic disorder, not a cardiac condition, and the doctor writes a prescription. After a time, Ann believes the medication helps a little, but she is still plagued with anxiety. Thinking that psychotherapy might help, Ann's doctor gives her my card. She calls immediately and makes an appointment. By the time she comes in to see me, she has been out of work for a month. She's still unable to face the long drive, and she doesn't know if she is going to be able to return anytime soon.

As a clinician in a solo, private practice, I'm always pleased by new referrals, and people with anxiety are my bread and butter, the bulk of my caseload. This is not surprising since anxiety disorders are the most common psychiatric conditions, according to the Centers for Disease Control and Prevention, particularly in developed countries.

In the United States, social isolation and the constant flood of information from the media create a breeding ground for anxiety. Isolation leaves people like Ann lonely and vulnerable to a host of psychological maladies including anxiety. The Internet and television news, in turn, present a steady stream of frightening stories—murder, sexual assault, even the risk of cancer-causing cleaners in our own homes. Americans worry about possible dangers lurking around every corner and frequently develop anxiety disorders as a result. Sometimes Boston, where I live and work, feels like a taut string, waiting to snap.

I meet with Ann twice a week for a month. Slowly, I piece together her story.

"My mom," Ann says, "was sixteen when she had me, and my dad was only eighteen. She told me that she wanted to have an abortion, but my father wouldn't let her. My aunt and uncle came in the middle of the night and took me away from my mom, and I only had one shoe on."

"Why did they take you from your mom?" I ask.

"She wasn't responsible. She was," Ann replies, "neglectful."

She goes on to describe the drugs and alcohol that dominated her mother's life, and I imagine baby Ann crying for hours in her crib without anyone comforting her.

As a child, she lives with her aunt and uncle and visits her mom and dad. Her stomach hurts frequently. Her head aches. She doesn't like going out of the house because she is afraid to be away from home.

Her parents split up, and her dad takes up with another woman with whom he has more children. Ann dislikes visiting him and his new family, but her aunt makes her go, saying, "He *is* your dad."

"Aunt Mary says hello," she remembers telling her dad when she is only five years old.

"So what?" her father responds. "Life sucks and then you die."

I picture Ann as a young child caught in the tight web of some longstanding family conflict. Every time she has to see her dad, Ann's stomachaches worsen.

At age twelve, she sneaks pills out of her aunt's container of Xanax, a highly addictive anti-anxiety medication. It doesn't take long for her to discover that drugs are the best escape from the anxiety. For the next twenty-plus years, drugs are her constant companions.

The anxiety begins again when she finally becomes clean. Since people frequently turn to drugs to numb feelings, the link between Ann's newfound sobriety and her renewed anxiety isn't surprising. It is a pattern I have observed before.

Ann's treatment progresses slowly. Many people have hurt her in the past, and she takes her time trusting me.

After Ann leaves her tenth session, I claim the comfy chair to decompress. The bright sun streaming through the window on this cold winter day does little to calm me; I consider the likelihood that I will soon receive an unwelcome call from her insurance company requesting a review of her progress. Health insurance companies might easily see twice-weekly psychotherapy—once the norm in the pre-managed-care, Freudian days—as excessive, particularly if the symptoms do not subside. But I need them to authorize and ultimately pay for continued treatment if I am going to be able to see Ann. They are footing the bill, and they *should* ask me some questions. Nonetheless, I always feel like I must assume the role of a supplicant during my telephone conversations with them.

Ann's return-to-work date adds more pressure. Over the weeks of her therapy with me, I have dutifully filled out the forms sent to me by her employer's disability insurer. *Can she dress and bathe herself on her own?* Yes. *Can she concentrate, follow specific instructions, and perform under stress?* No, I answer in all honesty. With a hefty co-pay of thirty-five dollars per session, Ann's disability check is as essential for continued treatment as is authorization from her health insurance.

Another month goes by. As Ann closes the door behind her after one of her visits, I reconsider the details of her case. The anti-anxiety medication prescribed by Ann's doctor works well for the majority of patients but seems less effective for Ann. The "gold standard" for the psychological treatment of anxiety is cognitive behavioral therapy. In its most distilled form, cognitive therapy maintains that thoughts influence feelings, and errors in thinking cause anxiety. In the world of cognitive behavioral therapy, Ann's fear of having a heart attack, evoked by her shortness of breath, is called catastrophic thinking and requires correction. Treatment then revolves around helping patients develop more accurate thoughts about their fears. Should Ann ultimately recognize that nervousness, not a cardiac event, produced her respiratory distress, a cognitive therapist would be very happy, indeed.

Many psychologists clearly identify themselves as cognitive-behavioral therapists, but I am reluctant to take on such a label. For me, the pleasure of the job lies in its creativity and flexibility, the freedom to borrow from different therapeutic schools of thought. Without a rigid adherence to particular form of psychotherapy, I listen to the patient with an open mind and tailor the treatment to her concerns.

Still, cognitive-behavioral therapy may be the best option for Ann, as research studies show that correcting erroneous thoughts can effectively reduce nervous responses. I turn to the National Institute of Mental Health (NIMH) for guidance. Cognitive behavioral treatment, I read, often lasts about twelve weeks.

Uh-oh, I think. I am at the end of my third month of treatment with Ann, and she's showing little improvement. I've certainly identified examples of catastrophic thinking, but maybe I haven't clearly described the cognitive errors. *Is it me?* I wonder. *Am I doing something wrong?*

I redouble my efforts. In Ann's next session, I suggest her fear of having a heart attack when she is short of breath might be catastrophic thinking. "Remember how you can be out of breath after running up the stairs, and that is perfectly normal," I remind her.

But Ann still isn't buying it. Something must be seriously wrong with her body—not her mind—when she cannot breathe properly. "Could it be a cancer?" she murmurs to me. "My mother died of cancer when she was in her forties."

Having faced cancer myself, I bristle at Ann's irrational fear. The illness left me with an acute awareness of my own mortality, knowledge I often wish I could escape. Maybe I envy other people's good health, but their unfounded fears of cancer and death try my patience. *Come on, Ann*, I think. *We're all going to die someday. Live a little*.

Perhaps reading the irritation on my face, Ann tries to show me that she is a good patient, working hard at getting better. "I always try to follow your suggestions," she nearly whispers.

Her diminished voice reminds me of her history—the neglect Ann experienced and her likely efforts to be a very good girl to earn her parents' love.

"I don't want you to think that I am not trying," she adds.

Regardless of favorable studies, cognitive therapy doesn't work for everyone, and it clearly isn't working for Ann. Invisible to most of the adults in her life as she was growing up, I understand then, Ann just wants me to listen to her stories. I wonder if my statements about thinking errors sound critical to her; I have treated patients before who reacted this way. Good care, I remind myself, requires flexibility. I recognize Ann's need, even if it doesn't follow the protocol. In the dance of therapy, she leads, I follow.

Nonetheless, I can't ignore the pressing realities: the health insurance reviewer, the weekly disability forms, and last but not least, my own sense of professional inadequacy. The comfy chair beckons. As soon as Ann leaves, I collapse into it.

Then it comes to me: the dodo bird verdict.

The Dodo in *Alice's Adventures in Wonderland* judges a race and decides to let all the participants win. "*Everybody* has won, and all must have prizes," the bird announces. In his 1936 article in the *American Journal of Orthopsychiatry*, the psychologist Saul Rosenzweig coined the phrase "dodo bird verdict" to point out that different psychotherapeutic approaches—with proponents who passionately and unyieldingly oppose one another—are equally effective in making patients feel better. Consequently, all of these techniques, said Rosenzweig, win the race. How then do patients heal? According to Rosenzweig and numerous researchers who came after him, good therapists share certain characteristics essential for a patient's improvement, particularly empathy and hope.

Empathy is easy. A patient like Ann arranges the facts of her life before me like pieces of a jigsaw puzzle. When the pieces match, coherence emerges from those irregular shapes. As I stand back, the puzzle comes together. Her thoughts and feelings have a logic of their own. I can readily imagine the feelings of a woman struggling to face anxiety that is no longer masked by drugs and alcohol; my bout with cancer introduced me to the experience of a full-blown panic attack—the tight chest, the pounding heart, the feeling that you can't get enough air into your lungs. These are the same symptoms that eventually led Ann into my office. My empathy for her is effortless.

Hope is harder. Ann has faced a lifetime of damage, inflicted by Ann herself as well as by other people in her life. She often tells me that all the drugs have destroyed her brain. She confesses with embarrassment, "I can't remember many things."

Some days the avalanche of adversity faced by my patients is daunting. Confronted with a full schedule of patients' hardships, I can feel helpless; I just cannot think of a thing to say. As I flip through my notes, I am surprised to discover how many people have come in for an initial appointment and never returned. *Don't they like me? Haven't I helped them, even a little bit?* Occasionally, it even occurs to me that I am not cut out to be a psychotherapist.

In these moments, I reconsider the meaning of hope and the work of psychologist Charles Snyder, who maintains that goals are central to hope. According to Snyder, an individual with hope has an objective. She imagines paths to achieve her aim and recognizes her own efforts will ultimately take her to her goal. Hope is an active process, the steps we take to create the life we want for ourselves.

I think about my years practicing psychotherapy: the privilege of listening to people dream aloud about the kind of life they want and watching their efforts to make it happen. Hope in a nutshell. I look to my patients for hope as much as they look to me. Their improvement is, in fact, my therapy. They give meaning to my life and keep my angst at bay.

"The brain is plastic, malleable," I finally reply to Ann. "People have strokes and recover. Individuals with brain damage improve. So can you."

I pack the cognitive therapy tools back in the box and stop trying so hard to "make" Ann better. I go back to what I think I do best: listening. Her stories pour out, conveying an urgency to have someone witness her life. I concentrate on Ann's face, and I notice her pause before she speaks. This hesitation conveys so much shame and embarrassment that her story about sexual abuse is exactly what I expected. I imagine that my quiet attention to her words feels like a downy comforter, softening the boundaries between us.

The existential psychiatrist Irvin Yalom writes, "It's the relationship that heals." Though Yalom's approach is out of fashion now, his words reassure me that I am helping Ann and the rest of my patients, too.

The deadline approaches when Ann's employer expects her to return to her job. On her own, Ann decides to practice commuting to her office with her boyfriend a few times before she tries to do it alone. Her return-to-work day arrives, and she makes the drive. Every day it becomes a little easier.

NIMH claims that "the behavioral part [of cognitive behavioral treatment] helps people change the way they react to anxiety-provoking situations." Pausing, I consider Ann's perseverance—driving her car in the face of anxiety rather than staying home. Perhaps the tools of cognitive therapy helped her after all.

I breathe a deep sigh of relief.

In the end, I cannot say for sure why Ann finally improves. But sometimes I do think of a particular day when she slowly raised her eyes from the spot on the floor that had seemingly captured her attention for much of the hour. Her eyes meet mine, and we both smile. She makes a funny comment about gaining too much weight, and I burst out laughing with an appreciative snort. I tell her that I sometimes shop at the bakery she visits. "Their cheesecake is delicious," I confess. We both nod enthusiastically, having a similar weakness for sweets. Ann asks me if I have any children. "A son who just graduated from college," I tell her. "He has his first job and an apartment." I think then that Ann is the right age. She could be my daughter.

Soon after this visit, Ann disappears for a number of months, as patients frequently do when they start to feel better. She resurfaces when her uncle is dying. After his death, she quits her job, saying that she is sick of the long commute back and forth to work. She tells me that she wants to spend more time with her aunt. But I start to worry that she is taking a few steps backward.

Ann, however, makes a number of changes in her life. She takes up figure skating again. She reconnects with an old friend who is planning a vacation to Costa Rica and wants her to come along. Ann's boyfriend offers to buy her the plane ticket for the trip.

I ask Ann to Google Costa Rica and see what comes up. Two weeks later she comes in and tells me she saw pictures of Costa Rica. The scenery is beautiful.

"I know it isn't heaven with angels and clouds," Ann says.

"But it makes you think about what heaven might be like," I suggest.

Eventually, Ann says she can't go on the trip because she is about to begin a watercolor class. "But I know that if I can think about it, even for just an hour, it is possible that I will get there one day."

When Ann leaves my office, I curl up in the comfy chair and glance at the *QE2* poster that she could see the first day she visited me. "For Once in Your Life, Live!"

I feel hopeful that for Ann these words are beginning to come true.

....

Ellen Holtzman, PsyD, is a psychologist practicing in Wakefield, Massachusetts.

ILLUSIONS OF WELLNESS

Katherine Sheppard Carrane

A therapist struggles with the unexpected death of a longtime patient who had seemed to be recovering from depression and addictions and making a new life for himself.

The moment I learned of his suicide was not what I'd pictured it would be. No middle-of-the-night phone call or knock on the door by a policeman. These were the scenes I had rehearsed in my mind, preparing myself. Few people would or could survive his risky behavior. So, over the ten years I'd known him, I'd become resigned to readying myself for bad news, anticipating that he would die, preparing to lose a patient whom I cared a great deal for. Ultimately, I wasn't asked to do anything but to know that he was gone.

I was surrounded by strangers on a train, late at night, in the dark, unforgiving cold of a Chicago winter evening. Heading home from the city to the northern suburbs, after my late day at work, I sat and spread my things out beside me as best I could, hoping no one would sit next to me. After talking and listening to a lot of new patients, I wasn't in the mood to chat or share my seat. I was back to work after a two-year hiatus due to some health issues and was still regaining my endurance for long days. I glanced at my phone while searching for my train pass and saw that I had a message from a number I didn't recognize. What if it was one of my children calling on a friend's phone or a new patient in my practice who might be in crisis? I hesitated for a split second, and then listened to the message.

It had been left by his former boyfriend, Jim, who calmly stated that he wanted to tell me that Ray had died at the beginning of the month. I listened to that message several times to make sure I had heard it right, as if my brain were fast asleep but vaguely hearing an early-morning alarm clock. I wasn't processing. Apparently the years of orderly intellectual preparation for his possible death had failed me. I wept, wanting the comfort of those strangers I'd so readily dismissed.

I sat in my daughter's room after arriving home and dialed Jim's number. Jim had been in Ray's life for some time, first as a lover, and then as a friend. I had met with him several times when Ray had been struggling with their relationship and they came in together for a session or two. He had been a kind man, staying with Ray through many a storm.

"Hi Jim, it's Katherine."

"Katherine, oh, I am so glad to hear your voice. I know it's been a long time since you've seen Ray." It had been two years. "We don't know what happened, other than he disappeared for several days and then we found him, unconscious, in the ICU of a local hospital. We—Billy and Alice and Moe and I—were with him when he died. I've ordered an autopsy. I'll let you know the results when I find out what happened."

Jim had always been in denial about Ray's struggles. For a moment, I was hoping my gut was wrong about Ray's death, wanting to believe that he had died of a natural cause, not by his own hand. I joined Jim in his denial and chose not to ask any more questions.

For ten years before I temporarily closed my practice, four o'clock on a Thursday meant I would see Ray. He was always on time no matter what his activities were leading up to his appointment. I had come to rely on his reliability.

He would sit in the small waiting room furnished with black chrome chairs that were nice to look at but not so comfortable to sit in. The chairs weren't unlike many of the people who entered the office, shiny on the outside but without the proper stuffing inside of them to hold the weight of their problems—people like Ray.

Ray was in his late thirties when we began our work together. He had been in plenty of therapy offices over the years. I wondered if he even noticed the stiffness of the chairs or if he had developed immunity to their discomfort. He had been referred to me by his psychiatrist, who was treating him with a cocktail of medications for post-traumatic stress disorder and addictions of varying sorts.

"Hey Kath, I have a referral for you," my old friend and colleague had said in the message he'd left me. "It's a guy I've seen for meds for a few years, HIV-positive, substance abuser, history of sexual abuse by mother and possibly father and by the therapist he saw as an adolescent . . . god-awful. Anyway, he is a really sweet guy, obviously has a lot of trust issues, but wants to work on things. Let me know if you want me to give him your name?"

This was my charge, to gain Ray's trust, to be like no one else in his world. I wondered, given all of these breaches, if trusting another human being was even possible for him. What's more, could I do this work? I made a deal with myself to try to be there for this man.

He was seeing a devoted internist who was treating him with drugs for HIV, which he had contracted while working as a prostitute for a time after college. The three of us would become his treatment team, until one of us would run out of steam, and then there would be only two, and then one. At times, new doctors were added to take the place of those who could no longer bear the weight of his acuity.

Enduring multiple traumas had not diminished Ray's interest in the world. "How are you, Katherine?" he would say. "Did you happen to hear the interview on NPR this morning with Anne Lamott?"

"No," I would say, wondering who Anne Lamott was.

"Have you read her latest book? If you haven't, you should pick it up; it's all about parenting."

His cooking skills were stellar. On many occasions, he would enter the office with a small, neatly folded brown bag holding a piece of scrumptious blueberry-lemon cake he'd made out of the *Moosewood Cookbook*.

One day, he revealed his passion for gardening. With dirt on his pants and under his fingernails, he entered the office.

"I have been gardening for twelve hours straight!" he said, showing me his sunburned arms and dirty hands.

When I wanted to know more, he explained that because he didn't have a backyard of his own, he would find plots of land in the city that were littered with garbage and weeds and adopt them. Often harvesting seeds inside during the winter months, he would plant a variety of flowering perennials, creating beauty in spots that would otherwise lie barren and desolate.

"I'm a bit of a squatter, I suppose," he said with embarrassment and shame in his voice. Using this moment to connect with the part of him looking for acceptance and encouragement, things he'd received so little of growing up, I replied, "That is extraordinary."

He gazed at me with momentary puzzlement and then, in a different voice altogether, said, "I'll take some pictures and show you my gardens."

Later he revealed his fear of being taken off to jail for claiming city property as his own. We spent time talking about actions worth prosecuting and ones that weren't so criminal. He laughed, "Yes officer, I am guilty of planting the hollyhocks, and the zinnias are my doing as well."

I was often lured by Ray's strengths. He presented as so capable, likeable, someone who could thrive in the world. This blindness of mine, avoiding the darker sides of Ray, didn't help either one of us.

One winter day when I opened the door to the waiting room, Ray's silence revealed that something was wrong. "Hi Ray!" I said, sensing his hesitancy to come in. He avoided my welcome, holding his head down and away. He sat on the couch across from me like a frightened animal beaten one too many times by its owner, crouching, with his head hung low. The tingling began in my lower stomach, then rose up through my chest and throat until my eyes stung. I had been blessed and burdened by this sensation since I was a little girl. When I was younger, and conflict was thick in my family, I relied on this feeling to know when to get myself out of the house. As a therapist, I tried to let the feeling guide me so that I could remain present in the midst of someone else's crisis.

He raised his face to mine after a long minute, revealing dried blood around his nose, his normally dancing warm brown eyes wiped of their expression. We both winced as he showed his broken face to me.

"Ray, what has happened?"

"It isn't good, Katherine." Managing to keep his hazy focus directed my way, he said, "I acted out last night . . . this morning. Well . . ." His voice trailed off.

"Are you, hurt?" I asked, grasping for a direction to go in.

"No, I'm not hurt. Well, no one really hurt me, other than me."

I learned that after doing crystal meth, Ray had had unprotected sex with over eighteen men the night before, for hours on end. He might have infected some with the HIV virus, or maybe he would contract syphilis. He had left the bathhouse early in the morning, seeing sunlight for the first time in two days, so he could go home to get ready for his therapy appointment. He hadn't wanted to keep me waiting.

"What were you looking for?" I asked, ineffectively.

"Connections," he said slowly and remorsefully. "Just connections."

We would eventually understand these spells to be dissociative states that left Ray in a trance; he couldn't put words to his actions. His acting-out episodes would catch me off guard at times, thinking he was well when he wasn't. These collisions into the depths of Ray's mental illness would jolt me into understanding the severity of his wounds. For a time, I convinced myself in spite of knowing his history that I would be a different kind of therapist to Ray, not quitting, withstanding the unthinkable, helping him in ways others had not. But as these self-destructive episodes accumulated, my resolve began to break into bits. Doubt seeped into the treatment. The consistency and comfort of our relationship, availing myself to him through his pain, threatened not to be enough in the face of the ravaging effects of his addiction and depression.

I tried a proactive tact. "Ray, what would have happened if you had called me before leaving your apartment?" I asked, after one of these episodes.

"I don't think it would have made a difference," he said. "I wanted to go. I shaved my entire body. That is my ritual. Then . . ."

I listened.

"I did, for the first time, think, maybe I should go home. But I didn't; I just kept walking until I went inside."

This was an opening I had not heard from him before, this possibility of change.

"Do you remember thinking about turning around and what that felt like?" I asked, wanting him to see this slight beacon of light.

"I do, I felt more conscious. I thought I could go home instead. But the urge was too strong, so I did what I always do." His voice was void of emotion as he told me this.

"Ray, where is your fear?" I said, with tears replacing the stinging in my eyes. "You could have died . . . Ray"—my voice breaking—"you could have died."

"Yes, I guess I could have." He looked up and noticing my broken face, he wept.

The longer we met, the more he revealed. The treatment did not proceed in a linear progression toward health. A few months into his treatment, he chose to leave therapy, claiming that he didn't want to get better. I had to admit, I felt a guilt-ridden sense of relief from the burden of worry about Ray.

"Katherine, thank you for everything," he said, "but I am not going to change, so I think I am just wasting your time."

"I don't think leaving right now is a wise idea, Ray," I told him. "We have only just started to understand some of why you do what you do to yourself."

He left anyway.

He returned several weeks later after numerous visits to a bathhouse for anonymous sex, sometimes with drugs in his system, sometimes without. "What was I thinking, leaving therapy?" he asked.

Later in his treatment, when we were in agreement that he was fairly stable, Ray again decided to try life without therapy. After a break of many months, I got a call from his psychiatrist. He told me that Ray was dying.

I called Ray.

"Katherine, they can't find out what is wrong with me." His voice was weak and scared. "I need to come in to talk to you."

Ray appeared frail and frightened in the waiting room. He explained that after he left therapy, he'd begun acting out excessively and fallen ill. He was told by his internist that he might not live. "Katherine, I don't want to die." I had never heard Ray utter these words.

Shortly after our talk, he was admitted to the hospital, where he had his spleen removed. It weighed over seven pounds. He recovered.

Ray had no conscious awareness of what led him to these acts. The emotional disconnections in his brain were rampant. This is how early childhood trauma can show itself. It can permeate every cell in one's brain, in each hemisphere, disconnecting circuitry meant to be soldered together through relational well-being. There had been no well-being in Ray's relationships.

Ray's relationship with his mother had been complicated. He was slow to talk about it. One week he might give a gruesome detail about their incestuous connection, only to return the following week having shut down access to those feelings altogether. An episode of acting out sexually often followed a discussion about his mother. This painfully charged relationship was what Ray needed to understand in order to begin to recover.

During one session, it became clear that Ray was in need of a car in order to get to a job located some distance from his apartment. "I suppose I could ask my mother to help me out. She certainly has the means," he said. To his surprise, she agreed under the condition that he visit her to pick up the monthly check for the car payment. He did so, entering the house he had grown up in. "I saw my mother last night," he said, entering the office in a tattered state. "I went straight to the baths from her house and used crystal meth. She made me feel so badly about my life."

He struggled to let others in his life. His familial relationships were riddled with pain and abandonment, connections and disconnections. His father had been a distant figure, dying when Ray was in college. He wondered if his father had been a closeted homosexual as he had a memory of waiting in the car while his father went to meet men in other cars. "Did you know what he was doing?" I asked. "No, not at the time, but I think I do now," he replied.

Ray had a relationship with one of his sisters, but it was complicated by what he perceived to be the normalcy of her life; she was married with children, financially secure. She would push him to do things he felt he couldn't, such as work regularly or pursue a master's degree. He visited her once at her home in California and spent the weekend on her couch, curled up in a ball, unable to move. "She doesn't get how really sick I am," he would say.

With a glaring scarcity of friends, Ray would spend days in his apartment alone. Though his fantasies had him at a plentiful table surrounded by friends and family for Thanksgiving dinner, in reality, he shied away from follow-through with others, preferring solitude, and spent holidays alone, holed up, eating takeout and watching old sci-fi movies.

Romantically, he had chosen men who were narcissistic and unable to give him love, reinforcing his theory that he was unlovable. After he was abused by these suitors, he was alone. Our sessions were a rare opportunity for contact with another human being. In his frequent visits to the bathhouses he felt as if he were spending time with ghosts.

After a long time without anyone, he had allowed Jim into his life. They had met at a recovery meeting. But after a playful romance, Ray began to push Jim away as their intimacy started to deepen.

"I've decided that Jim should just be my friend," he told me during one late-afternoon session. "I can't be physically intimate with him and he deserves that in his life, even though he told me things are fine the way they are."

"There are lots of kinds of intimacy, Ray," I said, somewhat panicked, as Jim was the only person whom Ray saw with any regularity, other than myself. "Could you continue to date and talk to him about slowing the physical part down?"

"No, I don't think I can do that," Ray replied. "I would really rather be by myself . . . really, it is much easier."

After much discussion, Ray kept Jim in his life as a friend. They would grow to be supports for each other. Ray began to appreciate Jim's presence and allowed some of Jim's friends into his life, attending events with them and cooking meals. These friendships seemed steady from the outside, but internally, Ray struggled with the closeness of love. He expressed concern that his friends would learn things about him that would drive them away. Often, he tested their availability by sabotaging the stability of things, disappearing and then coming home to confess his acting-out episodes to them. In spite of it all, they stuck by Ray. He began to notice this.

Throughout his treatment, Ray had been obstinate, not wanting to attend recovery meetings, not interested in psychiatric day-treatment programs, dismissing the need for twice-a-week therapy, ignoring signs that he could benefit from a halfway house. He'd let me in a little bit, and then close up, as if he were returning a book to the library just when he got to the thick of the plot. These were dark days for the two of us. I grew weary and wondered if I could maintain a connection with someone so wounded. His psychiatrist had decided that he could no longer treat him due to his risky behavior and lack of willingness to change. I was beginning to feel this way as well, although the deal I had made with myself, to be there for this man whom so many had given up on, stayed with me. I began losing sleep, worrying about Ray's potential to die on my watch. I took a stance. He needed additional treatment. I was carrying too much.

"Ray, I feel as if you are digging in your heels," I said one afternoon, exasperated. "We are going in circles, sparring with each other over additional treatment that could really help you. What is hard for you about going to a group meeting?"

"Well, I guess it's because of the therapist I saw when I was a teenager," he said. "He would make us sit in a group, the eight of us boys, and would ask us to come and sit on his lap. I would feel special when he called my name, but scared at the same time. I could feel his erection through his pants and I knew this wasn't right."

He revealed more to me about the trauma he had suffered at the hands of this therapist, who was supposed to be helping Ray heal from the sexual trauma he had endured at the hands of his mother, who was supposed to be his parent. I backed down and listened. "Ray, I am sorry this happened to you." He decided to try an AA meeting but sit so that he could see everyone in the room, facing the exit so he knew he could leave if he had to.

I am not sure when the shift happened; it might have been after his first hospitalization. Prior to that, he had come to a session after a two-day binge on crystal meth and anonymous sex.

"I told Jim about where I've been and what I've done," he said.

"What did he say to you?" I asked.

"He was angry, because I disappeared. Mostly he was scared for me. He told me I could die."

"Ray . . ." I began, my voice quieting.

He interrupted me. "I know I shouldn't do this because it hurts me, but the last people I would want to hurt are Jim, and . . . you."

"Ray, I know people in your life hurt you and no one did anything about it," I said, then continued, "If I continue to turn a blind eye, I will be just like them. Something needs to change. I can't continue to treat you if you continue to harm yourself this way."

He nodded.

"I think you need to be admitted to the hospital, to interrupt this cycle of harming yourself."

"Well . . . yes, I guess that is a good idea," he said. This wasn't the answer I had anticipated. He added, "I guess I have been screaming for help and you heard me."

I had been leaning back during this time in Ray's treatment, yet he was moving closer to taking responsibility.

He felt cared for by the inpatient staff. I visited him on the unit and sat with him quietly in his room. "I have never been taken care of like this," he told me. "My mother just wasn't able to be there for me. I think I need to spend less time with her."

After his discharge from the hospital, Ray came in one winter day, a traditionally hard time of year for him, and said, "I was going to go to the bathhouse last night, but I stopped myself. I actually turned around and went back home. I locked myself in my apartment. I didn't want to hurt myself!"

"What was different about last night?" I asked timidly, as if my question would jinx this significant change.

"I want to live, Katherine," he said. "Plus"—he laughed—"how could I leave the dog I was babysitting?"

After that session, I closed the door and sat in the uncomfortable waiting room chair, which shook as I wept. Wellness was budding. I was a bit surprised that it had shown up, finally, like an unexpected gift that came in the mail. I feared that what I had to tell Ray soon would undo the scaffolding that was holding him up.

I was having a health crisis of my own. While I finally had the answers that I'd been desperately looking for, I was exhausted. So I did what I didn't think I would ever do. I decided to close my practice of sixteen years so that I could catch my breath.

The previous spring, I'd awoken to find that I couldn't see out of my right eye. A black line ran down the center of my vision, leaving me weak and in unimaginable pain. Over the course of fifteen months, I'd met with three specialists, searching for answers to this mysterious illness. Finally, I was given a diagnosis that was far better than what I had been told originally, but, while I had continued to work through this difficult time, I was tired. Rest seemed to be the only way I would be able to regain my equilibrium.

Ray continued to feel better. One day, he told me that after weeks of preparation, he'd attended a Sexual Compulsives Anonymous meeting. "I can't believe I can sit with other men in a group, feel safe, and hear stories similar to mine." He continued to go and asked a longtime member to be his sponsor.

Another day, he told me that a young couple, Alice and Moe, successful filmmakers whom he had met through Jim, wanted to hire him to be their gardener at a studio they were opening near his house. He would be in charge of the grounds and given an unlimited budget to plant a rooftop deck. "I can't believe my good fortune!" he said, smiling through his tears.

He hadn't been able to work a full-time job in many years. His agoraphobia, drug use, paranoia, compulsivity, and depression had interfered with his ability to hold down a job for any length of time.

It was time to tell Ray of my decision to stop practicing. He seemed ready. He was launching into the world, as if moving out of the dorms and into an apartment. I wondered if his wellness was related to unconscious knowledge on his part that I had been sick. Had he gotten better because he knew I needed a break, or had the therapy helped to heal his deep wounds?

I often think of the last session we had together. He brought in a package wrapped in white paper. "I didn't know what to give you to say thank you, so Jim helped me put this together for you." I opened the package to find a book of photos of the gardens he'd planted.

"You know," he said with tears in his eyes, "you will never get rid of me." He laughed.

"Why would I want to, Ray?" I said. "Why would I want to?"

· · ·

Two years and three months after I last saw him, Ray left his apartment and went to the bathhouse to do drugs and have anonymous sex, to fall on his way home, to be found by a stranger and taken to the ICU, to be surrounded by his friends, who had spent days calling his empty apartment, before he took his last breath. I will never know if he would have survived longer if we had been able to continue our work together. I suspect he would have. I also believe that one's body can survive only so much before the breath runs out.

I learned of Ray's death six weeks after I returned to work. I had decided that I wouldn't contact my old patients to let them know I was back, as it seemed they had moved on to lives beyond our therapy days together. I have been left with the thought of what might have changed if I had called Ray. Would he have acted out anyway, in spite of what had become a meaningful relationship for both of us? He might have, eventually, as that is the nature of mental illness: it can creep back into one's life just when one's armor to combat it has grown a bit rusty.

I entered the cold, snow-covered chapel in one of the oldest cemeteries in Chicago. There were many people inside the small elegant stone space. I saw faces I recognized from Ray's descriptions and ones I didn't know. The quiet murmur of voices filled the room. I thought about the times I'd imagined he might die, alone, with no one to notice he was gone but me.

I approached Jim and hugged him.

"Katherine!" he said. "You made it!" Jim was a tall, good-looking man with chiseled features and lots of strawberry-blond hair. "Go and see Billy," he pointed to a friend of Ray's I had met once during his hospitalization, whom Ray had been living with for the past two years. "He has something for you, from Ray."

"For me?"

I found Billy. He hugged me and handed me a small white box. "He had gotten this for you after your therapy ended, but he didn't mail it," he laughed. "He didn't think it was big enough. I found it by his journals, and thought you should have it." He hesitated. "Katherine . . . Ray said over and over in his journals that you saved him."

Standing at his funeral, looking at the enlarged picture of Ray smiling, I had no words. He was gone. I was standing by his ashes. And yet it felt that everyone there who knew of Ray's struggles collectively understood that he should have died, over and over, years earlier. He had been able to stay on the earth a bit longer as a result of his work in therapy. A man with no connections had built them. His death wasn't a reflection of what had failed, but of the strong hold, even if momentary, that depression and addictions can have over those who valiantly fight them on a daily basis. He had relapsed. It had been after Christmas, after his birthday in late December, after New Year's. That night, he had gone back to a way of coping with his darkness that did not allow him to turn around or call a friend, actions that might have saved him from himself. Ray had decided differently the night of his death. The voices luring him into the shadows had been loud, drowning out his inner strength.

I opened the box and found a sparkling silver chain with an oval pendant hanging from it, the color of amber. "He told me after he'd ordered it that the stone has healing powers," said Billy. I put it on and smiled, wiping the tears from my eyes.

The service began. The priest spoke of Ray's love of dogs, friends, food, and flowers. Music soared and echoed through the small chapel where we huddled together for warmth on wooden pews. Friends spoke of his kindness. Ray was surrounded by love.

Before his final prayer, the priest told everyone to take a packet of seeds on the way out. I passed the basket and noticed the pink hollyhocks that graced the small envelopes. I held one of the packets along with the empty small white box in my hands. I carried them in my pocket for days afterward, reaching in to feel them.

I never planted those seeds, for I am a gardener in my mind, but not in actuality. The packet remains in my drawer at my new office, where I can be reminded of what can be.

I went into the studio where Ray had worked. It was a modern space, filled with light, movie paraphernalia, and people eating gourmet food. I approached a young woman behind the front desk; she was directing the stream of people arriving from the funeral.

"Excuse me," I said, "I am a friend of Ray's and I was wondering if you could take me to see the rooftop deck?"

"Sure," she replied. "Let me get the keys to the elevator."

She returned and showed me to the back of the large room, guiding me into a glass tube.

"It is kind of like Willy Wonka's elevator," she laughed.

We arrived on the top floor and she opened the door to the vast deck, covered in snow. I bent down to touch a planter that held dried stems of hollyhocks, ones I had seen in the book Ray had given me two years earlier, and as I watched the dried leaves flutter off of the dead stems, I said good-bye.

....

Katherine Sheppard Carrane lives in Glenview, Illinois, with her husband and two daughters. She is a staff therapist at Cathedral Counseling Center in Chicago and has a private practice. This is her first published essay.

STALKER

George Drinka

*While treating a ten-year-old with suicidal thoughts, a psychologist begins
to suspect child abuse. But after learning about the girl's fascination with
horror films, he begins to wonder if his young patient is instead the victim
of violent and graphic media.*

Curiosity, fear, and anger: these are the three emotions afoot
in a pleasurable if dizzying dance at the heart of a popular
and controversial cluster of media creations, the American horror
movie. In my work as a child and adolescent psychiatrist in
private practice, I have heard many children describe the details
of certain horror films with mounting excitement mingled with
distress, while denying their anxiety. Others have told me more
candidly of their passing through periods in their development
when they watched such films with fascination, especially when
encouraged to do so by peers. Only later did they find themselves
plagued with bad dreams or irrational preoccupations with
werewolves or murderous clowns, or slashers with long claws.

While curiosity, titillation, and excitement pull a child into
such films, these feelings often lead the viewer to spine-tingling
fear and paralyzing terror. Further, since the menacing stalker
at the center of such films is generally motivated by murderous
fury and anger beyond bounds, the child-viewer must taste these
emotions too. Media imagery performs its complex magic trick

with subtlety, rendering the horrific attractive within the child's rapt psyche.

In a traditional child-development trajectory, the child suffers from a certain amount of fear, often related to anxiety over the dark, associated with separation from the parent, most notably the mother who serves as consoler, counselor, and secure base. As the child grows toward independence and self-sureness, and the mother wraps her offspring in a skein of love and encouragement, the average child grows courageous enough to venture into the world armed with a desire to explore, many times casting off any cautionary tales offered by the parent. This step in child development, which springs from the vital emotion called curiosity, stirs the child forward in his development.

In our time, this is where the media tends to step in. As parental connections weaken, a trend occurring naturally, and sometimes sped along by parental distraction, the role of the TV and the media as a parenting figure has quietly strengthened. The notion of parents serving both as secure base and as imparters of comforting if cautionary messages has become more muddled. The plethora of media imagery that now meanders into our children's eyes and ears and lodges in their imaginations has grown more vivid, more convincing, more nettling.

The creators of media stories, in particular action films and horror movies, often are experts in tapping into the already mentioned medley of primary emotions—fear, anger, and curiosity—enticing our children with imagery that fills them with confusing yearnings never experienced before in such abundance in the history of childhood.

Specifically I am speaking of the child's inner world where fantasy and reality mingle. Even apparently healthy children until about the age of eight cannot readily distinguish between their fantasies and reality, between dreams and the waking state.

This is why many experts have posited that children aged eight or younger are especially terrified by grotesque-looking if clearly fictional monsters.*

Further, many normal-seeming children interpret images springing from the TV screen quite literally until the age of ten or eleven, and only vaguely realize that they are watching fantasies concocted by others. They fail to realize that much that frightens or lures them is only make-believe. This is not surprising since media images, even ones rooted solely in fantasy, actually step beyond the inner realm of fancy and enter reality since the child really hears them, really sees them on the screen. They imbed deeply in his or her mind-brain in the form of real memories. Hence after watching horror movies, children often wake in the night screaming and rush to their parents' bed for comfort.

The two key emotions elicited by the horror movie are curiosity mingled with its opposite, fear. This dyad exists in a strange tension and dances warily, if pleasurably, about the child. A third emotion, anger, usually to the point of murderous fury, is often cast out onto the other—that is, the villain, the terrorizer, the monster that haunts the horror film. Yet the child identifies with the protagonist, whose fear of the stalker must transform into a mirroring fury, a cool-minded hatred, in order for the villain to be bested and destroyed by the hero.

Lara was ten years old when she first came to see me because of suicidal threats. The younger of her parents' two daughters, she had begun to brood on death about five months prior. She had written many suicide notes and strewn these around the house, only to claim later that they were jokes.

....

* Joanne Cantor, "Fright Reactions to Mass Media," in *Media Effects: Advances in Theory and Research*, 3rd ed., ed. Jennings Bryant and Mary Beth Oliver (New York: Routledge, 2009), 294–96.

Her history revealed that her nuclear family had recently uprooted itself from Simi Valley in California. Her parents worked at an international banking corporation that constantly shifted its employees around the country, giving them ultimatums to move to other states or lose their jobs. Lara's family did as they were told and meekly transferred to our city, Portland, Oregon. Rather quickly, Lara, her sister, and their mother had all become despondent, then clinically depressed. And the father was laid off anyway. The mother, now the primary breadwinner, traveled tirelessly to other parts of the country, serving as a troubleshooter for branches of the corporation even as she struggled to put her depression in its place via therapy and medication.

With her father a corporate casualty and her mother on trips, Lara pined away for her friends and old haunts in "the valley," as she called Simi, and stopped going to school. When she began penning suicide notes, her parents grew alarmed and conveyed their girl, these notes, and their concerns to my office.

Lara was a pretty and pale-skinned little girl who looked marvelously much like a juvenile Morticia Addams. That is, she was a bit of a goth. Listlessly she slumped in a chair in my office and refused to make eye contact or even to speak. She disdained seeing me or anybody else, as she had made clear to her parents in tirades on the way to my office. Through her long silences and sneering pouts in our sessions, she conveyed this conviction to me.

Her concerned parents and I initiated once-weekly individual therapy with me as well as once-weekly family therapy with a social worker. As my patient seemed low on energy, was sleeping poorly, and brooded on suicide, I concluded it prudent to begin an antidepressant medication. This latter decision proved a blunder. First, Lara refused to swallow the medication. Then she overdosed. After a frantic night in an emergency room, she was briefly hospitalized in a psychiatric unit. Within a week she was discharged and returned to my care.

For many more sessions, she remained angry and grudgingly silent, and I began to perceive myself as a kind of bogeyman in her eyes, a fearsome figure she seemed to hate. "Why is she so resistant?" I kept asking myself. "Who am I to her?"

In my waiting room when I came to find her, she often would cling to the furniture and plead with her mom and dad to spare her the sessions. As they were insistent, she would enter my office with hunched shoulders, tears trickling down her face. Turning to the wall, she either screamed four-letter words at me or cried incessantly, "I want Daddy. I want Daddy."

In this anguished manner, many months crawled past. I suspected child abuse and explored this possibility with her parents, but we came up empty-handed. Eventually, despite the seemingly fruitless nature of our work, Lara began attending school again, was no longer writing suicide notes, and was beginning to sleep better. She even made a few friends at school. Her antipathy toward her new hometown and its denizens was beginning to melt.

My first true dialogue with Lara occurred six months into her therapy, after news of an earthquake in Southern California. The quake had demolished homes and schools and cracked apart a cluster of city streets, and Lara voiced her fear for the lives of her old friends there.

"I talked with Susie," she said, as if she had already told me all about Susie.

"Is Susie a friend from Simi?" I asked.

"Yeah, my best friend there."

"It must be hard to be so far away from your best friend."

"Yeah." She smiled wanly. "But with the earthquake, I'm happy she isn't dead."

"You must have been really scared until you talked with her."

"I was, but I'm still scared about aftershocks."

Between games of Clue and Othello, which we now played together, she began depicting an idyllic life in Simi Valley. There she had resided for more than eight years in the same house. Her aunts, uncles, and cousins lived within an hour's drive. She had attended a special school for gifted children and excelled in science and math. Vividly she recalled the local skating rink with its canned organ music, the drugstore with its pop machine, a homey pizzeria, and a fifties-style hamburger restaurant, all within an easy walk from her home.

"Now I understand," I said one day, "why you miss the valley so much."

"Lucky for e-mails and Facebook." She received daily updates on Facebook about her friends. "But it's not the same," she added.

Gradually she began to reveal pride over her father's logical abilities and her mother's capacity as a bank supervisor. She began to fantasize aloud about her hope to own an art gallery in a funky mountain community nearby. With much enthusiasm, she conveyed her wishes to sharpen her skills in school and in the social sphere. Also, she revealed her confusion about religion, a precocious topic for such a young girl.

Since many children in her local school were fundamentalists, she often fell into vitriolic quarrels with them. Her own belief in scientific principles like evolution and relativity seemed more logical and grounded in scientific data, she archly stated, as well as closely allied with the perspectives of her parents. Often, in games of Clue or Othello or Battleship, she would use strategies her father had taught her.

"He's a genius in these games," she cried one day. "He's good at logic and science too."

It was clear that she loved him desperately. Never did she mention that he was laid off and, while holed up in the family home and sending out resumes via the Internet, was growing more and more discouraged with himself.

It was only in the tenth month of treatment that Lara first broached the subject of Charles Manson. With a shimmer in her eyes she recalled the fact, well known to her but not to me, that upon the brow of a hill overlooking the sweet valley of her childhood there perched an ominous estate, the Spahn Ranch.

There, several decades before her birth, this dark and brooding figure had dwelt, she revealed. Though buried decades in the past, the Manson murders remained alive in the memory of Lara, her family, and community. In a manner characteristic of an adult patient free-associating to a dream, she recalled standing in a variety store in Simi Valley and witnessing a testy interchange between its proprietor, who was selling T-shirts with portraits of Charles Manson dyed into their fabric, and an irate customer.

"Why are you selling these?" the customer had cried. "He's a brutal murderer."

"He is not," replied the hard-nosed owner. "He's a religious leader."

"What?" stammered the startled customer. "What do you mean?"

"He was convicted not of murder but of conspiracy to commit murder. His cult followers killed Sharon Tate."

Lara beamed as she recounted to me this snippet, claiming that the proprietor was logically correct. Besides, the guy had the legal right to sell the shirts in order to make a buck in a capitalistic society.

"So who committed the murders?" I asked, unclear of the facts myself.

"The three girls he brainwashed," was her reply. "Don't you remember the story? Now they're locked up," she added smugly, "and someone threw away the key."

In the mind of this eleven-year-old girl, I glimpsed the outlines of a prototypal figure that populates the psyches of many children in our time. Vividly I could see the homes, the schools, the stores, and the playgrounds in the happy valley of Lara's childhood, which flooded her with warmth and nostalgia. Yet looming above this pleasant vale stood the brainwasher of American youth, the demonic Charles Manson, who had charmed gullible girls into performing acts of carnage and murder. Manson was an incarnation of this prototypal figure: the serial killer, the cult murderer, the bloodthirsty stalker. Many more have lived and thrived since then, some in films and TV, others in real life.

Interspersed with our dialogues on Simi Valley and Charles Manson, another theme slowly unfurled itself. Lara prided herself on watching certain horror movies on Saturday nights, often alone. Frequently she fell asleep in front of the TV, long before the film's end, its lurid images and ripping sounds drifting through the rills of her sleep, mingling almost certainly with her dreams.

It was only then that I began to wonder if the abuse from which I had suspected she suffered was not actual abuse by a living, breathing human being but rather trauma caused by media mayhem, media-engendered abuse. As there is some scientific literature that makes this point, I began to conjure the hypothesis, however provisional. Was it possible that the media, in a sense, was her perpetrator?

"Where are your parents when you watch these films?" I suddenly asked.

"In their bed, asleep. Mom especially is always tired."

"So they're okay with your watching these movies all night long?"

"They'd rather have me safe at home watching a movie than out with friends doing who knows what."

She loved to describe in vivid detail scenes from favorite films in which killers slashed beautiful faces. Bodies were lit afire. Bullets pumped into human flesh and set the bodies dancing to their tunes. Be these humans murderers or victims, their yowling in pain seemed delicious to her.

"Does watching these movies give you bad dreams or nightmares?" I asked.

"Never," she triumphantly said. "Or if they do, I use a technique I learned from one of them to overcome the fear."

"What is that?"

"In Bali, when people dream of anything scary, they believe it best to go with the fear and so learn not to be afraid. It works every time."

Enthusing, she launched into a description of the film that seemed the source of this pop psychology idea, the original *A Nightmare on Elm Street*.

Still dumbfounded, I asked again, "So these movies never frighten you?"

"Fear? Never! You see, I find them funny. They make me laugh."

"Why funny? Aren't they gruesome?"

"They're just plain funny to me."

She free-associated to another Charles Manson anecdote from her childhood. A boy in Simi called everybody he didn't like a Manson groupie. Whenever a teacher gave him a poor grade, he ranted about how the teacher was a closet member of the Manson cult. If not invited to a sleepover birthday party by a classmate, he described the party as a Manson cult orgy. Smirking impishly, Lara both disdained the boy for his peevishness and admired his quick wit.

I recalled our early meetings, during which the timid girl remained frozen, crying out, "I want Daddy," as if I were terrorizing her. I concluded that Lara, who now rambled blithely on about acts of cruelty by Manson groupies and blended these seamlessly with her loving descriptions of horror films, was revealing the underpinning of her own psychological life, her internal play space. Here fear and sadism, the terrified and the terrorizer, exchanged places from moment to moment. I wondered about her attraction to horror films and specifically to *A Nightmare on Elm Street*.

This film sets its sights on two teenage girls, Tina and Nancy, who struggle with a demented child murderer and burn victim who stalks his victims from beyond the grave, Freddy Krueger. Along with their boyfriends, Glen and Rod, they confront this prototypal stalker, who pries his way into the dreams of teenagers and slashes them to smithereens in real life. The story takes place in a world that on its surface seems normal: Elm Street, America. Yet the girls suffer from an affliction that haunts the lives of many American children: fragmented families, missing fathers, and distracted, even drug-addicted mothers. Further, the film dances around a strange and shifting truth about how fear and horror work as entertainment: fear exists in the mind of the individual, the person being stalked, where it presents itself as dreams of terror and annihilation.

As the film begins, frightening dreams of Freddy Krueger are buffeting Tina, but the dreams enter reality when Freddy murders her in a bloody sequence in her bedroom. Surviving this horror, Nancy eventually sets out to confront Freddy. Bravely she works to enter into her own dreams where Freddy dwells and there destroy him. Meanwhile, Freddy kills Rod in the jail cell where he awaits trial, as well as Glen, who falls asleep in his own bed before he can meet with Nancy to assist in her quest.

But at the story's center stands the searing fact that throughout this adventure the parental figures are missing or inadequate. Tina's mother and father are divorced; her father is nowhere to be seen. On the night of Tina's murder, her mother is out of town with her boyfriend, and Tina is shacked up with Rod in her parentless home. As for Nancy, her mother's an alcoholic, often inebriated and unable to parent. Her father, a police officer, has wrongly arrested Rod for Tina's murder and refuses to believe his daughter about her struggle with Freddy.

In summary, the story resonates with a troubling moment in the history of many American families, including Lara's: the moment when the preteen or teen realizes with a tinge of anxious insight that she lives in a family with a paucity of credible parents. They are distracted by their professional lives and their personal problems; they cannot offer the child a secure base. Because of these failures, the child enters a world fraught with dangers like abuse and molestation, kidnapping and even serial killers, as well as access to certain teen activities like drug and alcohol abuse, early sexual initiation, and a media world brimming with dark imagery and scary notions.

In sleep, the fearful child drifts into dreams, which twist and career in directions beyond her control. She awakes in the darkness petrified and shouting for her parents who rush in, flick on a light, and soothe her. Only then do the vivid images fade, but not totally. Though Lara denied suffering from nightmares, it is likely that she did. Probably they had escaped from her memory at the moment she awoke. Instead of speaking of them, she transposed her dream fears onto her descriptions of horror films.

In the fictional *A Nightmare on Elm Street* and in Lara's real-life experiences, we see children terrorized by horrendous menaces. Parents prove ineffective in both the film and in life. Lara's mother suffered from bouts of depression and, like Tina's mother, disappeared for days on end. When home, Lara's mother was inactive and tearful—a burden to her daughter, if anything—and not a protector. In this way, she was much like Nancy's mother, who lived in an alcoholic stupor. The stress laid on Lara due to the employment dilemmas of both her parents loomed large, undergirding her sense of living in a menacing world, a worldview further enforced by Freddy Krueger.

Yet the film also offered a voice to her fears. Like Nancy in *Nightmare*, Lara drifted from a position of fear, trembling, and self-harm early in our treatment, into a form of action, if bizarre in nature. By watching horror movies for hours on end, she steeled herself against fear. Concurrently, she adopted a nonchalant and cynical attitude toward both horror films and the Manson murders. She used the technique of flooding herself with fearful images to ward off her fear of annihilation and pretend to herself that all was well. She turned fear into jokes. She denied anxiety and terror and renamed them fun. A strange and worrisome form of fun.

Many American youth struggle to cope via similar techniques with traumatic events like the ones Lara experienced. Ironically, many of the traumatic events that Lara faced were not events at all, but rather ones spilling from the TV screen. Whether the images are based on reality, as in news clips or documentaries, or fictional, as in horror films, they enter the brains and psyches of many children through the senses of hearing and vision, and through imagination. They implant in their memory-fibers. And they jumble together there, TV imagery and reality melting down and annealing.

Humans store select memories in their cortices via the intermediary workings of lower brain structures. While certain actual events of little import are rarely encoded in the memory at all, others, horrific in proportion, such as incest or exceedingly violent trauma, are also often lost to memory. Amnesia shrouds such troubling events as a kind of self-protective mechanism. In an intermediary zone of experience, however, where events seem arresting but not overwhelming in terms of fear or annihilation, certain images gain entry into the memory banks in the cortices.

Interestingly, horror film imagery often finds its place in this intermediary zone. Many of the images seem to remain long active in the brain. In a study done at two major Midwest universities, large groups of undergraduates were asked about films that had terrified them.[*] Surprisingly, over 25 percent reported that the effects of watching certain horror films had persisted for over a year and were still present at the time of the study. They reported lingering worries about the films and their characters, as well as avoidance of certain situations, for instance swimming in lakes or the ocean for fear of the shark in *Jaws* or the clown in *It*. Quite a large number had been visited into late adolescence and early adulthood by nightmares and other forms of sleep disturbance. In short, watching horror films leads to symptoms of post-traumatic stress disorder in many young persons. Many of these symptoms can linger for decades.[†]

What is the process by which curiosity leads to fear? The answer lies in the magic of storytelling. A clever screenwriter and deft director pique the viewer's curiosity by portraying events in such a way that they seem vitally important. Often the protagonist is a young person with whom the audience identifies. In *A Nightmare on Elm Street*, the troubled teens live in divorced families, a scenario familiar to many Americans both young and old. In Lara's case, the parents remained together, but the family stressors had escalated to the ceiling.

The horror film further entices viewers by drawing them into an alluring world. The female protagonists are usually physically attractive and live in comfy middle-class homes. Elm Street is

....

[*] Kristen Harrison and Joanne Cantor, "Tales from the Screen: Enduring Fright Reactions to Scary Media," *Media Psychology* 1 no. 2 (1999): 97–116.

[†] M. I. Singer, K. Slovak, T. Frierson, and P. York, "Viewing Preferences, Symptoms of Psychological Trauma, and Violent Behaviors among Children Who Watch Television," *Journal of the American Academy of Child and Adolescent Psychiatry* 37 (1998): 1041–48.

a nice place, after all. The film's protagonist is warm, caring, courageous, curious, and willing to take a risk, all traits that embody an American ideal.

Next, the horror film fashions a sequence of scenes in which rising suspense flows into shocking actions. The most lurid sequences, such as the one in *Nightmare* in which Tina's body scrapes the bedroom ceiling as she bleeds to death or the one in which the burning bodies of Nancy's mother and Freddy scorch a hole in her bed before her corpse drops into oblivion, possess a certain palpable intensity and even dark beauty that forces their imagery into the viewer's memory. In short, suspense runs into surprise, and surprise flows into horrific beauty.

Such films, in starts and snatches of pictorial imagery, have certainly etched themselves into scores of thousands of American psyches, as the study mentioned above suggests. These half-remembered images must seep into the dreams of our children, as dreams are by nature visual, based on events, including fictional ones, experienced during the daytime.

A final word on anger: the child who experiences trauma and terror in real life also feels fury toward the parent who has failed to protect her. Yet such an emotion often remains unstated. Similarly, horror films resonate so well with so many youth likely because they can now experience through their choice of media fare their fury toward the world that's failed them. Lara's case illustrates this dynamic well. On the one hand, she idealized her father. On the other, she must have been furious at him and her mother for uprooting her from Simi and dislocating her to Oregon.

The medium of the horror film has penetrated so incisively into American families and minds that it has in too many instances supplanted in weight and import many other adult messages in our children's lives. No wonder certain shockingly inhuman acts, often sexual and violent, now seem commonplace to our children, for they are firmly implanted there and seem natural solutions to, or outcomes of, actual problems.

The recommendations that spring from Lara's case seem both simple and subtle. First and foremost, when parents make a decision to uproot their families, they must anticipate the deep and potentially damaging effects of this decision. As a corollary, when parents grow depressed, they must not deny the serious effects such depression often has on the emotional lives of their children, as reams of clinical studies have made clear.*

Finally, parents must break through their denial of any deleterious impacts of such media creations as horror films. While parents may feel pleased to have their children sitting in front of a TV screen, don't be surprised if your child awakens in the night with bad dreams and mounting fear. Don't be perplexed when your child voices fears of unlikely events like stalkers kidnapping people from their homes and torturing them. And don't feel alone in being angry at yourself for allowing such events to unfold.

But also don't be surprised when a child like Lara grows enthused over such films and clamors to watch many. He or she may have developed what mental health therapists call affective or emotional numbing, for the data here are crystal clear.† When a

....

* William Beardslee, Eve Versage, and Tracy Gladstone, "Children of Affectively Ill Parents: A Review of the Past 10 Years," *Journal of the American Academy of Child and Adolescent Psychiatry* 37 no. 11 (1998): 1134–41; Erin Tully, William Iacono, and Matt McGue, "An Adoption Study of Parental Depression as an Environmental Liability for Adolescent Depression and Childhood Disruptive Disorders," *American Journal of Psychiatry* 165 no. 9 (2008): 1148–54.

† N. L. Carnagey, C. A. Anderson, and B. J. Bushman, "The Effect of Video Game Violence on Physiological Desensitization to Real-Life Violence," *Journal of Experimental Social Psychology* 43 (2007): 498–96; J. Murray, M. Liotti, P. Ingmundson, et al., "Children's Brain Activations While Viewing Televised Violence Revealed by fMRI," *Media Psychology* 8 no. 1 (2006): 25–37; R. Weber, U. Ritterfeld, and K. Mathiak, "Does Playing Violent Video Games Induce Aggression? Empirical Evidence of a Functional Magnetic Resonance Imaging Study," *Media Psychology* 8 no. 1 (2006): 39–60.

child watches visually lurid, graphically violent footage over and over and over again, he or she often is prone to much anxiety, sleeplessness, and fear. Yet the child can also develop a degree of emotional numbing to the violence she witnesses, a cardinal symptom of post-traumatic stress disorder. Such children may be prone to not feeling empathic when presented with violence, either fictional or real.

When a parent becomes aware of either of these trends in the child—elevated fear or desensitization to violence—he or she must work both to diminish such contact with the media and to insert him- or herself more fully into the child's life.

In the case of Lara, working in concert with the family therapist, I recommended that the parents strive, if subtly and sensitively, to diminish such contacts with horror films. With the father unemployed and depressed, we worked both to impact on his depression and to deepen his connection with Lara. Via board games, preparation of meals together, his taking her to art galleries and nature walks, and his facilitating her homework, he and his wife began to move this girl away from her depression and concurrently the genre of the horror film, into other areas of teenage and family life that would prove more constructive, less mired in the toxic combination of curiosity, fear, and anger, in spine-tingling suspense leading to moments of harrowing horror.

....

George Drinka, MD, practices child and adolescent psychiatry in Portland, Oregon. After attending the Johns Hopkins School of Medicine and a graduate program in modern history at Oxford, he completed his residency in psychiatry at Yale and his fellowship in child and adolescent psychiatry at Boston Children's Hospital, a Harvard-affiliated facility.

He became interested in the subject of children and the media in the 1990s, as his young patients frequently referenced media creations in therapy sessions. The author of The Birth of Neurosis, *he has written numerous case studies and published many articles on these patients and their media fascinations.*

NO HOPE? DON'T BELIEVE IT

Sharron Hoy

A mother's rejection leaves a woman isolated and incapable of emotion, but in counseling, she begins to experience true feelings for the first time. Now, this registered nurse has a sense of purpose, and she's passing on her testimony of recovery.

I was in the emergency room, somehow hovering above my head, unresponsive, but aware of everything that was being said. The hospital staff transferred me to another bed and I could feel how limp I was. A doctor was doing compressions and I silently asked myself in disbelief, "Are they doing that to *me*?" I was cognizant of it but couldn't really feel it. When all the commotion stopped, a man's voice said, "There, we saved another DOA." I tried to figure out what the acronym stood for and was unsuccessful. My suicide attempt had been sidetracked. How could I have gotten to that point, where I wanted to take my own life?

When I was four years old, I sat on the porch outside of our little white house with my little brother and my mom enjoying the cool evening breeze. I gave my mom a hug. She just sat there like I didn't exist—as if I were a ghost she didn't know was there. Unable to predict when she would accept me and when she would reject me, I thought, "I don't like you anymore." My detachment from her created in me the inability to receive any connection or love from her. As I grew, I forgot about my early experiences, and I didn't remember that love, feelings, and a sense of connection to others even existed. I thought that feelings were pictures that we drew like happy faces. I didn't know that they were something inside us.

When I was a little older, my mom's attitude evolved into hostility. "Get out of here," she would say. "Looking at you makes me want to throw up. Get away from me; you smell. Go look at yourself in the mirror, and then you wonder why nobody likes you." I would spend hours looking in the mirror, trying to figure out what it was about me that was so rejectable. It was as if I repulsed her. Her comments set up a lifetime of thinking I was gross and stinky even after I showered. If I wanted to try something myself and I failed, she would psychologically abandon me, snapping, "You wouldn't listen to me. You had to do it your own way. It's all your fault. You made your bed, now sleep in it."

My dad worked long hours. We saw him for only an hour or two during the evenings. During grade school, my summer days were filled with baton twirling, tap dancing, and tumbling. On winter days, I took piano and ballet—all without any emotion or awareness of feelings. At twelve, I became depressed for the first time. Hating life was my new attitude.

I submerged my life into competitive gymnastics. While other kids were socializing on weekends, I was traveling to meets, which was fine with me. I saw my female coach as a surrogate mother figure, but she had a mean streak. She would say things like, "Put socks on; no one wants to look at your ugly feet," and, "You need to lose weight, you're a big fat pig." That type of verbiage became the new normal. All through middle and high school, I didn't have one friend.

I got a gymnastics scholarship at a college in Texas. On my fifth day, I did a dismount off the balance beam and bent my knee backward several degrees, tearing my anterior cruciate ligament. Although I didn't realize it then, this was the end of my gymnastics career. I came back the following year but I couldn't compete as well as before. I was fifteen pounds heavier and couldn't seem to lose the weight. The disdain I had for myself was overwhelming and my untreated depression worsened. I abused diet pills. When I contracted hepatitis type A, I called my mom and told her I was very sick and needed to come home, she said that I had to stay and finish out the semester. That type of unempathic behavior was habitual for her. The university wanted me gone, so they put me on a plane home without my parents' permission.

I lived a couple more years with untreated severe depression, hating myself and wanting to be off this world. However at age twenty-two, I read in *Cosmo* that there were pills that could help with depression. I went to the local mental health center to get some. The doctor gave me antidepressants, which helped immensely. They had me talk to this really nice lady. At first, I didn't realize I was in counseling and couldn't figure out why she was willing to talk to me.

It was in counseling that I started to experience feelings for the first time. I felt like Helen Keller when I realized these emotions had names. What a surprise, they weren't just pictures! I was experiencing compassion from another for the first time in my life. I'd never known that this side existed. Subsequently, I developed an attachment to my first therapist and saw her as a strong mother figure. I attended group therapy and developed short-term friendships for the first time.

In the meantime, I was working my first job at a convenience store. After a year, I was falsely accused of stealing money and was fired. Devastated, I thought that if I cut myself, that would take the shame off of losing my job. This was my first cut. I lied at the ER about what had happened to my arm and got thirty-two stitches. My therapist knew it was self-inflicted and seemed angry. She said that if I did it again she would quit seeing me. I never did it again for nine years so I could continue to see her. Although she was kind, I never really trusted that she wouldn't reject me. I realized I still hadn't deeply connected to another—ever. My depression returned.

Things continued much the same way until I was thirty. That year, I was sitting alone in a back pew at church waiting for a women's Bible study to start when the pastor's wife, whom I'd never met though I knew who she was, looked at me with eyes that intensely sparkled. She wrapped an arm around me, pressed her face against mine, and asked me to move up closer to the front of the church. Oh! What was this feeling that I'd just experienced—a virgin occurrence of connection to another human being? I thought somehow God had showed her how deeply in pain I was. I felt wholly known and yet accepted for the first time. The physical contact facilitated this connection because I never was physically close to anyone. This one-time experience woke me up to this feeling. In having this for the first time in my life, I began to feel the loss of it.

Paradoxically, I spent the next twenty years trying to recreate the feeling of connection through cutting myself. I experienced some convoluted thinking that cutting myself might somehow bring about the type of relationship I craved. As a result of the cutting, I was inaccurately diagnosed with borderline personality disorder (BPD). According to the *Diagnostic and Statistical Manual of Mental Disorders*, a diagnosis of BPD depends on the patient meeting five out of nine criteria; I met only one: self-mutilation.

As tenuous as the diagnosis of BPD might have been, it preceded me wherever I went. Mental health professionals were wary and thought poorly of me even before we met. In general, clinicians try to avoid working with people who have BPD because their lives and relationships are chaotic. Borderline clients will love you and then hate you. They can be manipulative and destructive. Clinicians' reactions to my case were no exception. The label created the very opposite of the connection I longed for. I wanted so badly to be taken care of, especially by a mother figure. Yet this longing was overshadowed not only by rejection from mental health professionals but also by a much, much stronger need to keep to myself, one of the hallmarks of avoidant personality disorder. This label, a much more accurate description of my illness, described my avoidance of people and social situations out of intense shame, embarrassment, and fear of rejection.

Fantasy became my coping mechanism and further solidified my avoidance; the reality of connecting with another was much too frightening to pursue due to the many years of rejection and thoughts of myself as disgusting. Cutting was the perfect setup. I created a false scenario in which I believed cutting would prompt a mother figure to want to take care of me. I pretended over and over that she was compassionate and concerned while helping me. I imagined that she was holding me and keeping me safe. She would attend to my cut with great carefulness. I would dream that she would brush the hair out of my face, looking at me with warm eyes and a loving smile. Thus, my needs were being met, at least in my imagination. The responses I normally got from my real mother were not warmhearted but considerably icy. She had a limited ability to mother me because she was profoundly self-referential and had no empathy. My needs were not important to her. She probably didn't even recognize them.

When one fantasy lost its effectiveness and became boring, I needed new content, thus another severe cut. I cut long, wide, and deeply, penetrating fat cells. At first I would go to the ER and tell a fake story as to how the cut had happened. The day I got caught doing it on purpose the feeling of loss was so overwhelming. I was so desperate for the connection that I deliberately cut a tendon in my ankle and had to have surgery. I did this by slicing my tendon little by little. All of a sudden my foot fell and the muscle bunched up in my leg. That was frightening. However, I thought it had to be severe enough to elicit the concern I craved, even though I couldn't accept it from anyone real. I cut myself every month or so for decades. I stopped going to the ER to get sewed up because the cut provided relief but then the doctors became abusive to me, yelling at me rudely and degrading my personhood. I felt as though I didn't have a right to live, breathe, or especially have anyone be concerned about me.

My first therapist quit seeing me after ten years, saying that if she continued, she would be enabling me to keep cutting. I was devastated. I had always been sure she would ultimately reject me and now she had, further solidifying my inability to trust anyone. After six months without being assigned a new therapist, I called the mental health center and complained. A supervisor saw me. When I inquired about why it took so long to get a counselor, he stated that no one else would take me. After that, I went to see private therapists. I went through six therapists during the next ten years due to my inability to trust. Also during this time, I was seeing the pastor's wife monthly for Christian growth. The deep sense of connection I felt to her had created a desire to see her for individual meetings. I had asked her to meet with me and she was willing.

During that time, I was pursuing a master's degree in rehabilitation and mental health counseling. Despite my continued difficulties, I wanted to be just like my first therapist, helping others in pain and showing people compassion when they hadn't experienced it. A professor once told me that manipulation results from a strong need for connection coupled with a stronger fear of making that same connection. One motive for manipulation is to hide one's needs from others. It would have been horribly embarrassing to make my fantasies known, so I never explained my destructiveness. Cutting had some degree of manipulation in it by trying to have a mother figure be concerned.

Eventually, my Christian friends and the pastor's wife became frustrated with my cutting and with me. They thought that since

I continued to cut, I was letting Satan take over my life. They accused me of not wanting to get better. Clinicians became exasperated with me and their anger established my reputation as someone who had no hope for recovery, only management of symptoms; then again, probably not. I believed that I had no connection to anything or anyone on earth, and I became very depressed. Even the people who were hired to help me rejected me. I had no reason to be here on this planet.

I met a therapist in grad school who used holding therapy, a type of attachment therapy that continues to be controversial. The idea behind it was to help build trust and get the patient's developmental needs met. One can't grow developmentally unless one's needs are met at each stage. Since I had been arrested at an early stage, I was curious and strangely drawn to this type of work and decided to try it. Also, I craved physical contact immensely. During our first session, I was terrified. I was sitting on a couch. She was sitting in a chair across from me, wearing a light pink sweater and jeans. She said I had to ask to be held; she wouldn't just do it. Holding had so much shame attached to it. I was afraid that being that close to someone would cause rejection. I couldn't even say the words "Hold me." Instead, I would say, "Can we do that thing?"

The first time was petrifying. My hands were pressed tightly over my face. I had gross muscle shakes. I couldn't breathe in and I couldn't blow out because I was afraid my breath might smell bad. I was suffocating. I quickly pulled away to breathe. I felt intense shame. Did I repulse her? Did I make her want to vomit? Did I stink? On and on I thought about her reactions. However, when I went home, I had hope for the first time. I was so happy.

The holding experience, which happened when I was forty-two, was the start of a very frightening five years of therapy. After the first year, I became more comfortable with being held, but I was still scared. During the course of therapy we worked on stopping the cutting and dropping my belief in the BPD diagnosis, as she would comment over and over that I wasn't borderline. We also went through the criteria for BPD so she could prove it to me. I realized through therapy that besides depression, my accurate diagnoses were reactive attachment disorder and avoidant personality disorder. As I released the much-entrenched identity of BPD, I became very angry at the diagnosis I'd been given. That is when I became fervently opposed to slapping such a prejudicial diagnosis on someone without ample consideration. I wonder if clinicians realize how deeply it affects people when they so flippantly make diagnoses. When my therapist moved away abruptly, she left me half-baked, but I had experienced incredible relief and some healing with the holding therapy. However, I still had to work on my depression.

Over the years, I had been hospitalized about twenty times. My depression affected me physically so much that simply moving my body and lifting my arms became arduous. I see depression as 90 percent due to brain chemistry but sometimes brought on by disturbing emotional situations. My childhood experiences were a prime setup for severe depression. My first psychiatrist, however, never really did much to address my depression and rarely changed my meds over seventeen years. At the local mental health center, I would get kicked out of groups with an explanation that I didn't understand the material being discussed. But I felt my being asked to leave had more to do with my honesty about what I saw going on in the groups. I confronted a therapist in group therapy for telling her client to find healthier friends. I was her client's only friend, so she had been talking about me. She was advising her client to dump me. Finally at forty-four years old, due to my rejection by the mental health center, I decided to look for private psychiatric care and be completely free from the center.

The first new psychiatrist I saw had my records and refused to lift the "severe BPD" label. Although I was honest with her, she believed I never told the truth and that everything, including my reports of suicidal feelings, was a manipulation. My depression worsened and I became severely suicidal. I researched on the Internet how much of each of my meds I would have to take to kill myself. I was surprised that it would take so much. Oddly enough, amitriptyline, the medication my dog was on to treat separation anxiety, is lethal in relatively low doses. When I discovered that, I called my vet and asked if I could have more since it was inconvenient to drive to his office and get it so often. The receptionist gave me a big bottle. As it took only 1800 milligrams of amitriptyline to reach a lethal dose, I now had enough of it on hand. However, I was feeling ambivalent about killing myself.

When I saw my psychiatrist, she asked if I had suicidal feelings, as she did in every appointment. With my head and eyes down due to shame, I quietly specified that I had 1800 milligrams of amitriptyline. She replied that she wasn't going to play games with me. She apparently didn't believe me and thought I was trying to manipulate her. I was filled with intense shame and hurt. I respected her intellectually and also saw her as a surrogate mother figure. Yet again, I felt so rejected. The humiliation was overwhelming. I wanted to disappear.

A few days later, I woke up at two in the morning and turned on my bedside lamp. Hans, my little gray and white schnauzer puppy, was being treated for a hot spot. If this problem is not treated, dogs can scratch down to the bone. My dog was on the bed scratching the spot on his skin that was already deep; I was afraid it was going to get worse. I said to myself, "I can't handle this shit anymore." My desire to be invisible and off this earth was so overwhelming I couldn't take one more thing. I looked at the bottle of amitriptyline that was sitting on the table. I thought for a minute about taking them, and decided to do it. I took a small handful of the amitriptyline. I felt disgusting as usual even though I wasn't dirty, and didn't want to be found that way. I bathed and put on clean clothes. I then took the rest of the pills. I had never felt such a penetrating sense of peace in my life. I always thought it would be scary, but it wasn't. Quickly, I fell asleep.

I woke up in a dark ICU room with a breathing tube and another tube that was very black protruding from my nose. I found out later that it was charcoal that was being pumped into me. Charcoal absorbs some poisonous materials in the gastrointestinal system, reducing toxicity. Apparently, my mom had had some sort of intuition and had forced her way into my house with my brother, breaking my bedroom window. That was rather odd; she never liked to come and visit me.

My psychiatrist strutted in to my hospital room and said something I found very strange. She said disdainfully, "You almost killed yourself."

I thought, "Well that *was* the idea." She still thought I was being manipulative. It was the first time I had made a suicide attempt and the incredible peace that I experienced made it really easy to want to do it again. For about two years, I was driven to recreate that sense of peace, and I often thought of suicide, a mentality that put me at greater risk. Appointments with my psychiatrist continued to be turbulent. I liked her because she was smart, but I often felt that she completely rejected me. She ended up leaving town and moving her practice for personal reasons. I was distraught and relieved at the same time.

I'm from a sparsely populated state in the West where there is a shortage of psychiatrists. I saw a new psychiatrist who moved to the region from California around the same time my previous psychiatrist left. He had no idea of my reputation. For my first appointment, I wore long sleeves so he couldn't see the scars. I was so afraid that he was going to rebuff me. However, I felt as though I wasn't judged and that he just wanted to help. That was refreshing.

I never brought up that I used to cut or that I had a suicide attempt. We just conversed about my depression and medications. With my previous psychiatrist, when I had tried to tell her what meds had worked for me in the past, she dismissed my ideas. The new psychiatrist changed my meds as I wanted and created a combination that put me in remission from my depression.

Though I wasn't depressed anymore, I continued to have incredibly low self-esteem. At the age of forty-seven, I started working with another therapist. It seemed as though we weren't accomplishing anything for a couple of years, but I noticed that my self-esteem had greatly improved. Did she know what she was doing after all? She described her approach this way: "Recovery is in the doing in life, not in talking about life." She got me busy accomplishing small tasks. She identified that I had my own resources such as my intelligence and tapped into it by having me use my brain; her approach eventually included supporting my idea of going to nursing school. Having a narcissistic parent, I had been deprived of reflection and feedback, which is so necessary in developing healthy self-esteem. In contrast, my therapist provided mirroring and highlighted my accomplishments. This allowed me to believe in them and internalize them, and empowered me to take ownership of my achievements. She said that self-esteem comes from becoming skillful and gaining mastery.

Now that I was at last in remission and no longer cutting, I keenly realized the loss of twenty years. After getting my master's degree, I worked for a year as a child therapist in a residential setting before deciding to go to nursing school. It wasn't going to be easy. The long-term depression had severely affected my hippocampus, which plays a critical role in memory. The suicide attempt had also caused some damage by depriving my brain of oxygen for too long. I couldn't catch on to concepts quickly anymore or remember much, without tremendous effort, such as what the recent lecture had been about. That made school very difficult. However, I made it through and passed my licensing exam as a registered nurse.

Upon graduation, I applied for nursing jobs everywhere, including at the very mental health center that had rejected me as a patient. I decided just to let it play out because I didn't know what I was supposed to do with my life. Several years earlier, I'd finally lost my Christian faith after being rejected by my Christian friends and the pastor's wife. I still had my belief in God and hoped there was a greater plan and we humans weren't just running around like little rats in a diabolical experiment.

I gave an excellent interview at the mental health center and was actually hired. I was elated and thought my life's purpose was playing out. I had worked seven days when the director of the large mental health center learned who I was. Monday morning at 8:15, she called me into her office and announced that they had to let me go. When I asked her why, she asserted that I was in my probation period and she didn't have to have a reason. My supervisors were surprised because I had been doing an exemplary job. The very people who treat the mentally ill apparently did not believe in recovery.

I went through an existential crisis. I had applied to work at the mental health center because I knew I could bring hope to people with mental illnesses by demonstrating that recovery is attainable. I was perfect for that nursing job because not only was I an RN but my master's degree was in rehabilitation and mental health counseling. I was devastated and just didn't understand the turn of events. However, at a deeper level, I guess I expected it.

I was hired for two jobs in nursing homes, but I didn't think that was where I belonged. Neither did the employers. Saddened and feeling defeated, I started thinking that I wasn't supposed to work as a nurse. But I still hoped there was a plan for my life. My self-esteem had a giant notch cut out of it; I was questioning my purpose. I contacted an agency that provides personal care and nursing services to people in their homes. I thought that I could work as a personal care attendant. They just happened to have a job opening for a nurse helping people with severe mental illnesses. I couldn't believe it! I was so thrilled. I took the job and am thoroughly delighted about it. My typical day consists of filling med boxes, taking phone orders from physicians, and assessing the clients. In order to keep healthy enough to work as a productive nurse I have to take my meds as prescribed, have my own therapy once per week, and stay connected with my friends. Walking my dogs daily also helps with keeping me from getting depressed. I never had a significant other but maybe that can be in the future.

There are some key parts of my treatment that helped me recover. My first therapist made the sessions safe enough that I could become aware of my feelings and put names to them. People have to know that emotions exist and feel them before they can learn to deal with them effectively. I successfully attached to her, which helped me with my detachment issues. She also taught me about the defense mechanisms that I used the most, one being projection. Realizing that I displaced my feelings on others was crucial. For example, I saw myself as disgusting, but I was unaware of that and thought it was other people who thought I was disgusting. Knowing that took away a lot of fear I had toward others and helped me be around more people instead of just hiding away from them.

Another huge aspect of my healing was the holding therapy. I believe I got those maternal needs met so I could grow and move on with my life. I no longer needed the cutting and the surrogate mother fantasies. Holding therapy also helped me be able to be physically close to people without tremendous fear and avoidance.

Finally, the key to overcoming my depression was finding the right medication combination. Unfortunately, it took several years to find it. I think people deserve remission from depression and should not stop looking for a successful med combination until they find it. I measure my depression on a scale of zero, which means suicidal, to one hundred, which means complete remission. For me, anything under ninety is reason to keep looking for the right medications and doses.

As I continued to heal, my energy was no longer consumed with getting my basic psychological needs met or constantly thinking up ways to kill myself. I needed to find my talents. Pursuing vocation and finding meaningful purpose greatly helped with self-esteem and gave me a reason to get up in the morning.

My recovery, from what clinicians and I branded a "no hope" situation, is proof that recovery can occur—even for the sickest. To get that truth out, I am working at the local Mental Health Advisory Board trying to spread the word about recovery and reducing stigma. I designed a slogan that we have put on bumper stickers, microfiber cleaning cloths, and water bottles. In bright yellow letters over black it announces, "Caution: Treatment for mental illness can cause recovery."

I no longer crave a mother figure's attention, have given up my fantasies, and have stopped my cutting. I have been in remission for five years now. Clearly, my inaccurate diagnosis and branding with a bad reputation negatively skewed mental health professionals' behavior toward me. Their prejudices led to rejection, kept me sick and even put me in danger. My life proves that recovery is achievable. Maybe every one of us has a purpose after all, even those of us who believe we have no reason to be here on earth.

....

Sharron Hoy, RN, works as a psychiatric nurse and with people who have physical conditions. She is the author of Workforce Expansion: A Rehabilitation Model for Clients with Major Depression. *She has a master's degree in rehabilitation and mental health counseling, and serves on the Mental Health Advisory Board in Billings, Montana.*

CAME DOWN A PERSON

Ella Wilson

Plagued by shame and convinced she shouldn't be alive, a young mother finds herself pressing a broken cereal bowl into her arm while her children play in the other room. Can a generous art therapist's unconventional techniques bring this woman back from the brink?

M y therapist got off the bus with a backpack, a box of matches, and a shovel. She walked toward me smiling the kind of smile that they don't teach at therapy school. It was a golden Saturday at the end of June, and what we were doing was far beyond the realms of normal therapy.

Two years ago to the month, I had slit my wrist. It was a Tuesday afternoon and my almost-four-year-old was playing downstairs in the office with my husband and my eighteen-month-old was barreling around the kitchen floor with a spoon and the dog. I was up to my amygdala in Klonopin and unmanned misery and I was trying to cook dinner. Nothing was right, but I had no clear sense of what was wrong. This had been a long-standing problem. The more depressed I became, the more anti-anxiety medication my psychiatrist suggested I take. So I did. But one can become too unanxious. Unworried bordering on careless. Careless bordering on reckless. Reckless bordering on dead.

I drifted in a haze around the kitchen, trying to find anything to pass off as dinner. I found cereal and tofu and had some vague sense that I could combine the two with hot oil to create something crunchy and nutritious.

Over the years I have tried more ways to escape this misery than one hopes for in a lifetime—from Western remedies to Eastern medicine to ideas that neither hemisphere is willing to claim. But nothing has ever shifted the sense I have that I am not supposed to be alive. And when existing feels this foreign and hopeless—like getting off a plane in Nairobi to realize you have forgotten to pack your legs—dying does not seem like the bad idea that most people think it is.

In fact, when you look at your perfect, smart, chubby, bright nuts of children and all you see are small people who will eventually realize that life is just one sadness after another; when you look at the man you moved four thousand miles to be with because the very sound of his voice, the glimpse of his mind, made you excited to breathe, and see only a five-foot-ten Jewish male who walks too loudly; when you wake up in the morning with a painful shock that you are still here; when you feel nothing but sorry for everyone and everything, especially yourself, then death seems welcome, prudent even.

And so, as I rushed around the kitchen cooking dinner, which may have looked to an observer more like a confused lady slowly picking up and putting down the same items again and again, I dropped the cereal bowl. Corn flakes and china shattered and I shooed the toddler out of the way. I picked up the pieces of bowl and took them toward the bin. I stood with my foot on the pedal, a large shard of china in my right hand, sharp edge in the early evening light, and I stopped; everything came together and it looked an awful lot like nothing. I held the bowl over my left wrist and paused. Then I slashed it across the skin; I thought it would make a scratch. It didn't. A deep, dark world opened up on my arm. The blood looked black. It was coming from a deeper well than anything I had ever seen before.

The first time I tried to kill myself I was twelve. I tied a woolen scarf into a slipknot and hooked it on the back of the bathroom door. I placed the noose around my neck and I let my legs go loose. The scarf tightened. My face felt big and my eyes began to bulge. My knees grazed the reed matting of the bathroom floor and the edges of my vision went black. The screws of the hook cracked loose, splintering through the wood, and I knew I was in big trouble. I had broken the bathroom door.

What made possible both of these incidents was my sense of disconnection. At twelve I did not feel a part of my family, I was not one of my peers, I was not of this world. Suicide felt like a logical step. If you were a corporate lawyer who found himself at a modern dance retreat you would leave. I would.

Brené Brown, a research professor who has spent the past decade studying vulnerability, courage, and worthiness, tells us that nothing unravels connection like shame. A feeling that there is something wrong with us, something so wrong that if other people saw it they would no longer love us. Such a feeling makes it hard to connect to other people, to connect to ourselves, to connect to life at all. And shame can slip in easily when we are young. When we believe what we are told about ourselves. When we are dependent on our parents—who we realize only later were just a couple of people trying to make it through the day—for our sense of who we are.

When a parent criticizes a child, the child does not think: Fuck you! as an adult might; rather she thinks: Fuck me. And when a parent hits a child, she does not hit back, rather she tunnels that force inside her small body and turns it into a reason that her parent is perfect. The result of the ghastly equation being: there must be something very hittable about me. And when a parent abuses a child, the child does not tell the parent to get off; the child goes very still, the child sends parts of her soul away to protect it, the child burrows inside herself and hides her knowledge that this is wrong. The child is confused. The child is ashamed. The child is not so much of a child anymore.

It is in these moments of fear and misunderstanding that your cosmic rightness, your belief in the sky and earth, and the cellular confidence you were born with, are blindsided. A dark spot begins to grow inside you, an ink spill you want to keep hidden, a shameful stain that pushes you and the world in opposing directions; and the very thing you are a part of, life, begins to feel like the enemy. The string that connects all of us to the universe and each other is loosened and you are suddenly less than sure that this whole thing is such a grand idea after all.

Every time we fall in love or make a friend, hold someone tight or choose a muffin, get pregnant or buy new underwear, paint a room or eat a sandwich; every choice we make to stay, to treat ourselves as valuable people, to connect more and more with this thing that can end only in loss, in death, loneliness, holey underwear or shit; every time we choose connection, we are risking loss. But every time we do not choose connection, we are ensuring it.

We all have dark spots, some small—something between a sneeze and a tickle; some huge—like water reservoirs that supply whole towns: dark, deep, and on the outskirts. Some of us laugh too loudly and say mean things, some of us start fights. Some drink in the morning, others have a lot of cats, some go to doctors looking for answers, some hide in the bathroom and vomit up their dinner, some eat only white foods, some cut their arms and legs, some run marathons, others just stop focusing their eyes and wait.

I grew up far and alone on the Yorkshire moors in England. There were no other houses, no other people, just my parents, trees that lay close to the ground at the insistence of the wind, and sheep dotting the landscape like boulders. But my loneliness was not the place's fault.

Some children are born belonging to parents who belonged. Their mothers hold them and in those arms rests a generational knowing, a sense memory, of what it is like to be held. Their backs and heads and hearts send messages to one another, messages of safety and love.

And then there are the rest of us. With parents who did not know caring, parents who despite their fierce love cannot provide safety, parents who no matter how hard they try will never be whole or kind. No matter their intentions they are fated to deliver every message with an undercurrent of anger or hatred, indifference or carelessness, coldness or power.

My mother had grown up in the 1950s in London, in Germany, in Blackpool, in Bahrain, with an uncle in the English countryside, on U.S. Air Force bases, on her own, in the back of a car when she was twelve with an airman on top of her, with too many sisters, a mother who never smiled, and a father who drank. She had been abandoned and left for living. She wanted something different for me, but we cannot give what we do not have. She aimed for love and can hardly be blamed for missing; she had known only the opposite of holding and safety and was trying to fill in the rest for herself.

There are obvious abandonments of children, and then there are the smaller abandonments. My mother did not leave me on a doorstep. But when my father was diagnosed with cancer and

I cried and she told me to shut up, she abandoned me. When she looked at my changing teenage body and touched it and said, there is something wrong with you, she abandoned me. When we saw my father's dead body and my legs buckled and she told me to grow up, she abandoned me. When she insisted I sleep on my dead father's side of the bed, when she told me I was her best friend, when she told me about her sex life, when she flirted with my boyfriends, when she wouldn't let me close the bathroom door, when she asked in surprise how I ended up fat when she had had a twenty-one-inch waist at my age, when she spent so long drying between her legs with a towel in front of me that I thought I must be mistaken, when she told me somebody asked her if she had children and she said no because she forgot about me, when she sat and watched me bathe. By the time she died I was already left.

After I slit my wrist the cut became infected with MRSA and I spent two weeks having surgeries as vancomycin pumped through my system intravenously and the doctors tried to save my arm, my life. Through this time I was largely alone, except for a nurse on suicide watch. My husband stayed at home and tried to hold all the love and needs and spaghetti and baths that two small children require. And even when he did visit I was beyond being visited. There are places out beyond connection and I was in one of them.

For thirteen days a black woman sat next to my bed. A different one every eight hours, but always black and always a woman. These women were kind. Some were silent, others wanted to talk. Some texted, others fell asleep. But if they minded they did not show it. Hully, Martha, Nana, Gloria. Jamaica, Guyana, Haiti, Ghana. One at a time they washed me. They moved me gently, they lifted my arms and scrubbed my armpits, they gave me a flannel to wash between my legs, they soaped my back and rinsed me off.

One by one these women asked me if I went to church. I told them I did not. They asked if it was because there was not one nearby, or if it was because I worked on the weekends. Was I was too busy with the children? But one question never occurred to them.

"I don't believe in God," I told Patricia.

She looked at me, unflinchingly.

"Child," she said, "that's why you're here."

I did not believe she was right, but I had an awful sense that she might not be completely wrong either.

I had been a proud atheist for over thirty years. But I was a lopsided believer, the kind who believes in so much, just none of it good. I thought this was what an atheist was. I didn't believe in God; I didn't believe that there was anything after death other than black and no way to see it. I didn't believe in fate, energy, connection, or spirit. I believed in what I thought were the hard and fast facts: there is nothing here you cannot see, there is nothing before or after life, we are alone, anybody who believes any different is stupid. It seems I had drifted beyond atheist into the realms of cynic, from where it was but a short hop to full-on Prophet of Doom.

But for a self-professed unbeliever I believed an awful lot: I believed that I was not supposed to have been born. I believed I was the wrong child for my parents. I believed there was something intrinsically wrong with me that made me a nonviable candidate for life. I believed there was something dark inside me that I had to hide. I believed I could survive only if I was completely merged with my mother. I believed that I had to be on the second or sixth step of the staircase when the dining room door slammed. I believed things were my fault. I believed I had to eat foods in pairs: two apples, two bananas, two pieces of bread in case they got lonely in my stomach. I believed I had to use the toilet twenty-six times before I fell asleep. When my mother had cancer I started crossing my chest every time I saw an ambulance, a hearse, a cemetery. When my father had cancer I believed I had to use six paper towels in the hospital bathroom. When he died I began cutting my food into tiny pieces and eating two pieces an hour throughout the day. When my mother died, while I was pregnant, I believed my fetus was her reincarnated.

I spent a hell of a lot more time believing than most practicing Christians do. Everything I did was built on magical beliefs, spiritual hiccups, and soul-destroying thoughts.

When my then therapist found out I had slit my wrist she fired me over the telephone. Nothing gets rid of people like a suicide attempt. It seemed she was not made for this kind of thing; she suggested I find someone who was. The problem with that was that I had no idea what "this kind of thing" was. The closest I could come to it was: me.

I have been diagnosed with bipolar II, borderline personality disorder, anorexia, unipolar depression, generalized anxiety disorder, and treatment-resistant depression. These have been countered with Paxil, Effexor, Remeron, Klonopin, Xanax, Prozac, Zyprexa, Seroquel, Abilify, Lexapro, Celexa, Chinese herbs, electroconvulsive therapy, hypnosis, leafy greens, fish oil, vitamin B12, St. John's wort, group therapy, light therapy, talk therapy, cognitive behavioral therapy, dialectical behavioral therapy, eye movement desensitization and reprocessing, and acupuncture. But none of these things helped. There was no way they could. You cannot fix someone who does not feel connected to the idea of living with a pill, any more than you can fix a car without wheels by filling the washer reservoir with blue liquid.

The only way to come at a problem of this magnitude and confusion is not with sense; it is not with reason or science; it is not with pills or lists, electrodes or clever sayings. A problem of this scale and unnameability needs to be met with nonsense, with moonshine and malarkey. With magic and oracular thinking. Insanity meeting insanity.

I found a new therapist through my husband's therapist, whom I had in turn found for him. It is living in New York that makes sentences like this possible. She was an art therapist, which was not necessarily what I was looking for, but since I was pretty far beyond looking for anything other than a way out it seemed as good a choice as any—and after seven years of people nodding and smiling at me and suggesting I try holding an ice-cube instead of wanting to die, the fact that this woman owned a hot glue gun and a creative mind seemed like it could only be a good thing.

The first time I met my new therapist I did not know she believed in fairies. I did not know she would give me tarot cards as a birthday present. I did not know we would go night swimming together in a lake in upstate New York. I did not know that one evening when I was noodling around near the edge of safety she would text me, "I love you so fucking much you have no idea!" I did not know she would hold me for hours while I cried. I did not know we would set fire to things I hated and grind the ashes into the earth. I did not know she would come to my house and remove all my dead mother's underwear from my drawer and throw it in the garbage. I did not know I would tell her things I had never told anyone. I did not know she would understand what they meant. When I walked into her office for the first time I saw only that she was smart and tall and unfazed by my apparent condition, and that she had the same jeans on as I did. I saw in her face that she had not always been happy. I saw that she had woken up in the wrong places and bargained with God. These are things crazy people can sometimes spot in each other. I was glad for that at least. It is hard to lay bare one's hopeless soul to someone who has only ever lost a cat and shops at Lands' End.

She did not yet own a shovel; that would come later.

At first we met twice a week and when that did not seem like enough we added a phone session and when phone sessions did not feel like enough but I couldn't make it to Manhattan she came to Brooklyn and we sat on park benches. This may sound like a lot of therapy, but when hours feel untenable and bridges look like good ideas seven days can be an awfully long time.

But it was more than the regularity of appointments that weighted the scales of my soul. This therapist was not treating me like another client. She was doing more for me than therapists did. And this did not scare her. She was wonderfully unafraid to like me, to love me, to share her story with me, to walk down the street with me, to want me alive, to care for me. And this lack of fear on her part vibrated as she held my hands and smiled into me. We can do this.

In the beginning I did not know that she too had been abandoned in innumerable small ways. There had been an unstable mother, an absent father, religious communes, too many hands, drugs and men, deaths and fear. And as she sat across from me and shared with me her losses I saw her glowing with gains.

This woman was not a nodder, she was not a professional therapist in the bad sense of the phrase; what she was doing nobody could have taught in school. She was a connector. She did not leave me in my pain and sadness, she brought her own out to the moorlands that howled with wind and nothingness and sat down across from me. She offered up her fears and devastations as anchors. Her scars made her a believable hero. She was just the kind of woman who might change someone's life.

. . .

One month out of the hospital I began to tell my new therapist the stories I knew about myself. The stories I had told every other therapist I'd ever had. But we do not always know our own stories. She took the things that I had given other mental health professionals as the reasons for my lack of commitment to life and she handed them back to me wrapped in a new understanding. She asked me questions that at once made no sense and at the same time knocked my lungs clear with truth.

Like a criminal who subconsciously wants to get caught I was leaving clues everywhere. And like a loving Sherlock Holmes, she pieced my stories and scars, tears and hurt together and came to conclusions I could have spent a lifetime missing. In these conclusions I found both devastation and relief.

She was the first and only person to name my experiences as abuse. Emotional abuse. Sexual abuse. The first time she did I hung my head over her wastepaper basket trying not to vomit.

At that moment I had never felt more like dying but underneath the familiar urge to cease existing bubbled something different, I won't call it excitement, but somebody had heard what it was I didn't even know I was trying to say with my scarred legs and sewn-up arms, with my preference for hospital over home. Death over life.

"There is nothing wrong with you," she announced one day and I thought she had somewhat missed the point of me as an entity.

"There is nothing wrong with you, there never has been. You have just always thought there was, but there isn't! There's nothing wrong with you!"

She said this last part with an unrepressed joy that frightened me.

When you are underweight and covered in scars it is hard to believe you were born whole and lovely. It is harder still to look around and see where some of the wrongness you believe is your own may have seeped through your skin and into your heart.

But this woman gaily abandoned the diagnoses I'd been given. She threw out the stories I told her about myself. She rejected who I thought I was. She taught me some things should be left for dead, I just wasn't one of them.

Two years later the scar ran up my left arm, puckered and lumpy where the flesh had died and been brought back to life with blood flow and hope. I wore shorts and flip-flops to walk down the hill to meet my therapist.

I had driven to a retreat center in upstate New York a day earlier. The things I needed to let out felt too big for the confines of the city, with its slices of sky and wall on wall. The things I had been carrying around needed endless air and open sky. I could not loose this material upon Manhattan. Moreover, I did not trust myself to reveal these things to anyone and then walk out onto streets that roared with traffic forty-five minutes later. I had explained this to my therapist unaware that the disclosure would result in the plan we had together hatched.

The place we had chosen to do this work was a place where people come to meditate and do yoga, and while we would be doing neither—instead flying under the radar and embarking on a singular spiritual adventure—the ground at least felt prepared for the kinds of things we carried.

And so it was that I had spent a summer's night alone in a cabin in the woods, furiously writing and drawing and painting and gluing and trying in any way I could think of to get out all of the stuff I for too long thought of as my own.

The next morning, when I saw the brand-new shovel resting on my therapist's shoulder, I felt a sense of relief. You do not bring a shovel unless you are serious.

That night we dressed in black. And waited until everybody was asleep. I went into the bathroom and stared in the mirror for too long as if I were high, then I took a black pastel crayon and drew a cross on my chest. Something about aiming for the heart. Something about X marks the spot. Something about giving in to ritual and nonsense.

We packed up the drawings and writing I had done, images of pain and sadness, pictures of my body naked, my body invaded, exposed and broken, vicious images of what it felt like to live in a skin that does not feel like your own. Drawings of my mother's body that I knew too well, her body sewn up with cancer, her body dead, drawings of things I had no words for. And everything I had written, all the words I had been carrying around like a cloud of shame, making my life faraway and unseeable. We put it all in a backpack and walked up the pathways of the retreat, past trickling streams with little Buddha statues and meditation gardens. We crossed over a blank meadow toward the pitch of the woods. At the corner of the field a small opening led to a pathway in and with a flashlight we felt our way over stony ground and small rivers deep into the forest.

We had surveyed the woods in the daylight so we would know where we were headed by night, but sunshine cannot prepare you for darkness. Earlier we had skipped over rocks and rivers, pushed thorns aside and felt the sun dapple us. We had found a huge tree with a trunk that could bear what we would bring it later. I had sprung up the tree, into the branches; flip-flops to the wind I had climbed into the light, held the bark and waved down. This was to be the place. But night changes everything. We steeled ourselves against the black. Mosquitoes hung in the airless woods and nothing made a sound. We tripped and leant toward the spot that in the light had seemed like the spot and she handed me the shovel. I felt suddenly shy. I had never dug a hole to bury years of misery and shame in before, let alone in front of someone else. I was not sure how to start. But there was something about this woman, which doesn't even seem like quite the right word for her, as it makes her sound like a normal person. A woman with long hair and a cellphone, which she was, but to me she felt like so much more. It was this much-more-ness that she had shown me of herself that made the strangest things possible.

Because every time she did something like this, something she absolutely did not have to do, I felt unabandoned. And not just by her, but by life, by the universe that was allowing us to do this.

And I began to dig. Soon the very work of digging chased my embarrassment away and sweat ran down my forehead and bugs caught in my hair. She stepped back and let me hole. I dug into the mud and rocks. I raised the spade high and thrust it into the earth. I footed the tread with all my weight and sunk it deeper. Then on my knees I pulled rocks out with my hands. Shoulders shaking with effort, I dug further until the time to stop arrived.

Without speaking she handed me what it was I had brought to leave behind. I placed the drawings in the hole, carefully at first, until I had piled everything I had and then my hands took over, my animal, my cells that knew time, that had been fish and wolves and rain and leaves. In that moment I came alive in a different sense. I felt the pull of gravity and the push of time and I was a part of it, I have never been gladder to be included. And with that I shoved soil on top of shame and packed it down. I know I was speaking, then shouting. I told the earth what I no longer needed. I told it I knew it could hold for me what I no longer wanted to hold myself. I told it to stay put. I thanked the forest floor for its vastness and giving. I thanked the earth for its size and acceptance. I said things to that patch of earth that I have never said before and may never say again. Turns out soil is a good audience. And then it was over. All that was left was a pile with a big rock on top of it. We stood and looked at it until it wasn't time to do that anymore, then we gathered ourselves and walked out of the forest. I cried with my past at my back, even bad things can be missed. Following the river across the field we walked down to the lake, flat beneath the open sky. The smell of water was cold and black and we lay on the small strip of sand at the edge, uniquely aware of the two sides, the earth reaching deep beneath us, and the endless sky dotted with stars that evade time's reach. Somewhere a frog was making the sound of a donkey. The moon was high behind us and the stars shot across the night.

In that spell of stars and quiet it was simple: everything that had ever existed came from there. If I believed in the big bang like any science-fearing atheist did then I had to believe that in that flash, in that split and fury, in that violent birth: I was there, you were, so was my dog, your mailman, all of the Harlem Globetrotters, birds and feathers, lions and claws, leaves, rain, mud, hope, love, fire, hearts that beat, hearts that fail, moss, sand, rocks, and teeth.

This was a leap for a nonbeliever like me. To feel the eternity of it all and my place in it. Connection had never been a possibility for me. Now it was elemental.

Nobody can save anybody else's life—it is not theirs for the saving— but this person who lay next to me on the ground had come awfully close. Where life, people, and the things that happen when they get together had somehow pushed me toward nonexistence, this woman had drawn me closer. She had unabandoned me and taught me to unabandon myself. She had met me out on the bleak moors I had grown up on. She had smiled at strange times and heard things I did not know I had said. She had come at me with life and magic. Curiosity and prayer. Heart and soul. She had graced me with her heart and held me close with protective anger and fierce love. Obliquely she had turned my spirit toward itself and gently introduced it to the magic of the universe. With a gentle hand she had taken away the broken bowl and replaced it with things that nonbelievers nonbelieve in. Not once did she give up or look down. And that is how on the clearest of nights, with the sand at our backs, we flew up amongst the light and dark of it all and I came down a person.

....

Ella Wilson grew up on the Yorkshire moors in England and moved to New York in 2002. She has been writing nonfiction for the past twelve years and received her MFA from The New School, where she won the chapbook award, in May 2009. Ella has published work in several anthologies and is currently working on a collection of personal essays titled Existentially Challenged: A Merry Romp Through Illness, Depression and Death, *which is making her very happy. She lives with her husband and two daughters in Brooklyn.*